THE
TRANSFORMED
CELL

NOV. 1 1 1992

THE TRANSFORMED CELL

Unlocking the Mysteries of Cancer

Steven A. Rosenberg, M.D., Ph.D.
and John M. Barry

G. P. Putnam's Sons
New York

G. P. Putnam's Sons
Publishers Since 1838
200 Madison Avenue
New York, NY 10016

Library of Congress Cataloging-in-Publication Data

Rosenberg, Steven A.
The transformed cell : unlocking the mysteries of cancer / Steven
A. Rosenberg and John M. Barry.
p.   cm.
Includes index.
ISBN 0-399-13749-1
1. Rosenberg, Steven A.   2. Oncologists—United States—Biography.
3. Cancer—Research.   I. Barry, John M., date.   II. Title.
RC279.6.R67A3   1992   92-11864 CIP

Printed in the United States of America
1   2   3   4   5   6   7   8   9   10

This book is printed on acid-free paper.

For ALICE
BETH
RACHEL
NAOMI

—*S.A.R.*

CONTENTS

FOREWORD

In science, most significant efforts start with a question, and in a way, this book did as well.

About three years ago a friend, hearing me talk about my work, asked me, bewildered, "How do you find new treatments? Do you just take chemicals off the shelf and try them?" The questions were posed by an intelligent, inquisitive woman I had known for years, whose background was in the arts but who clearly had no idea how medical research was conducted. The naïveté of her question stunned me.

Lack of understanding can easily lead to misunderstanding, and science today often seems under siege. If so little is understood about how medical research is conducted, how can rational opinions be formed about issues such as the role of animals in research, the reliability of scientific information, the unpredictable pace of scientific progress, the need for public funding, and the social and ethical concerns surrounding the development of new medical technologies?

Unlike the arts, the conduct of science often bears little obvious relationship to everyday experience. Accounts of new scientific or medical advances that appear in the media present them in their final form, with little understanding of how the results were achieved. Many people eager if not desperate for the benefits of modern medical research feel increasingly alienated from science they find incomprehensible. Scientists, whose activities appear mysterious, often seem cold and detached from the implications of their findings.

I felt guilt in taking any time from my research to write this book. But it seemed so important to try to explain how scientists conduct medical research that I decided to attempt to explain it through my own experience seeking new treatments for patients with cancer. I approached John M. Barry, a writer whose talents I admire, to join me as a partner in this book, to help make the descriptions of the science understandable and, hopefully, interesting.

I did not keep a diary and had to rely on my recollections, enhanced by my laboratory notebooks of experiments, my scientific papers, and interviews with many of the participants in this story. The account is as accurate as such an imperfect method allows, except that I have changed the names of the patients to protect their privacy.

Medical research is an adventure. This book recounts one such adventure—an attempt to solve a mystery that causes the deaths of millions of innocent people each year—and through it, the fragile undertaking that is medical research.

Steven A. Rosenberg, M.D., Ph.D.

On the Verge of Mysteries

January 1991

It is 5:30 in the morning and I am at work. Already the hospital has begun to come to life, and a few hours from now two patients, Suzanne Marotto and Robert Antrim, my colleagues, and I will make a kind of history. Ms. Marotto, thirty years old, is exquisitely feminine with the grace and innocence of a deer. Oddly, her suffering has made her more innocent rather than bitter, and she has told me confidently this will be the year of her miracle. Mr. Antrim, forty-two, has a nine-year-old daughter. I have a nine-year-old daughter.

A few minutes ago I checked on them without waking them, making sure several procedures had gone properly, making sure their blood had been drawn at 4:30 A.M. so the test results would be available for rounds at 7:00, making sure that nothing untoward would interfere with what my colleagues and I have worked to bring about for months—years really.

I sip my coffee. A sip is all anyone can take. The coffee came from the nurses' lounge; they make a pot in the evening and leave it on a hot plate all night. By this time it is rank.

I think for a moment of all that I have learned in the last fifteen years. Too much of it is about the ways of the world, more than I want to know. But I have also learned that immunotherapy works against cancer.

Immunotherapy is far more than simply a new drug. It represents an entirely new approach to treating cancer, one completely different from the established modalities of surgery, radiation, and chemotherapy. Immunotherapy stimulates the patient's own immune system to attack the disease; the body's natural defenses can be made to devour cancer cells just as they devour invading bacteria.

The approach is still largely experimental, but we have treated many patients who have failed surgery, failed radiation, and failed chemotherapy, and who had only months to live. We have given many of them more time, maybe years more. And some of them we have cured.

But immunotherapy has as yet only tantalized us with its promise. We have made it work for only a few specific kinds of cancer, and even then we do not know which patients will respond to the treatment.

The experiment we are about to embark upon marks an effort to break out of this stalemate and to rewrite the rules under which medicine may work.

My colleagues W. French Anderson and Michael Blaese and I are about to alter the genetic makeup—the essence of all life—of Mr. Antrim and Ms. Marotto in an effort to cure their cancers. We are at the National Institutes of Health in Bethesda, Maryland, where the most sophisticated scientific advances are applied to treating patients; the concentration of scientists and resources here makes NIH unlike any other place in the world.

In two earlier experiments, the first in history, we cautiously inserted foreign genes into people to test the system we had devised. The first experiment simply demonstrated that our procedure did get a foreign gene into men and women and was safe. The second experiment tested the system at the next level by trying to show that gene therapy could help two patients with a genetically simple but rare disease—so rare that there are only about half a dozen victims in the United States.

This is different. This gene therapy experiment is no simple test of a system; it has direct, practical applications for the way we treat cancer. We identified cells in the two patients' immune systems that could attack their cancers, took those cells out of their bodies, and grew them into large numbers in the laboratory. We then inserted a gene into those cells that we hope will make them into viciously effective killers of cancer cells. Now we are about to infuse these transformed cells back into their bloodstreams.

Unless this new gene changes the way Mr. Antrim's and Ms. Marotto's bodies function, they will probably die before these words are published.

They are very different people. Miss Marotto is attractive, upbeat, and sensitive to her looks—to her lipstick, her earrings, the turban that hides her naked scalp. Forty small tumors are growing on her body and this cancer, this lethal metastatic melanoma, is a time bomb that could explode at any moment in a vital organ and kill her. She has endured many operations, chemotherapy, radiation therapy. All this has worn down those close to her, worn down her friends until it seems that they, but not she, have quit. Her grace hides her tenacity.

"People tell me I'm so strong. They say it sarcastically, like they're throwing it in my face. Like they hold it against me." She finishes speaking and presses her lips tightly together. It both puzzles and angers her that she can endure the strain but her friends cannot. A moment later, as if she does not want to be different from her friends, she denies her strength, adding, "I cry. I'm afraid."

Mr. Antrim also has melanoma. One tumor, the size of a large grapefruit, obtrudes from his thigh and has almost doubled in six weeks. If we cannot soon control this thing growing in him, it will burst through the skin. It will not be long before it kills him.

He is visibly uncomfortable here. Originally from South Carolina, he lives in a mountainous area of Virginia on a lake and tells me, "I'm not a bed-lying man."

The nurses meet his medical needs but seem to give him less attention than Ms. Marotto, with whom they identify more easily. They find him a little different, a little disturbing, with his black hair combed straight back in the style of a fifties teenager, tattoos on his arm, which he says he applied himself, and his ill-trimmed Fu Manchu mustache. Perhaps they find him a little frightening. In appearance, he seems to have a meanness, like one of the bitter and insular Southerners in James Dickey's *Deliverance*. I don't sense that meanness in him. He seems more like a wild creature

---

who in captivity grows lethargic, stops eating, and dies. One almost feels that any extended stay in the hospital will itself kill him.

I am desperate to get this gene into these two patients. Today. The politics of gene therapy, the need for approval from different regulatory bodies, is one of those complexities of the world I have learned about, and it has on occasion transformed me from a scientist and a doctor into a fierce bureaucratic infighter; it has left me weary, weary and angry, and I want to end these fights. Only making this experiment a fait accompli will do that. I want to act today. And even now I fear something will go wrong.

Almost immediately something does.

At 7:00, on rounds, I visit the two patients in the Intensive Care Unit for the second time this morning and examine their test results.

Mr. Antrim has a hematocrit of 16—indicating major internal bleeding, enough to kill him.

A nurse says he just vomited and it was rust-colored—another symptom of internal bleeding. A roll of panic twists my stomach but . . . Mr. Antrim looks at me, wishes me good morning, seems well. He could still be bleeding to death but . . . I quickly glance at the other numbers.

His potassium is 8—at that level his heart could stop at any instant.

I relax. Mr. Antrim cannot be experiencing the kind of sudden and total disintegration these two entirely unrelated threats to his life indicate. There has been contamination of the test, I am certain. A nurse drew the blood from the central line placed into his subclavian vein: The IV fluid must have contaminated the blood sample.

More disturbing than the contamination was the inattention of Mr. Antrim's nurse to the results. Anyone can make a physical mistake and inadvertently contaminate a sample, but this kind of mental error cannot be tolerated in our ICU. I call the head nurse aside. She explains that the nurse is new and promises to talk to her and watch her closely.

I order a second test to be done immediately, and order that the blood for the test come from a separate vein puncture. Later the results come back normal. What a way to begin this day.

The mistake reminds me of my first day in the laboratory in graduate school years ago, when I found my professor, Guido Guidotti, at the sink washing glassware while his technician was performing a complex task at the workbench. I asked him why the technician was not washing the glassware. "Because," he replied, "I always do the most important part of the experiment, and in this experiment the most important thing is the cleanliness of the glassware."

Therefore I decide to oversee the most important remaining part of this experiment. After rounds I watch the technicians harvest the cells with which we will treat Mr. Antrim and Ms. Marotto. They have been growing in dozens of one-liter bags filled with nutrients. The technicians are using a centrifuge to spin down the cells and extract them from the nutrient. Once the cells are concentrated in a saline solution, we will return them to the patients' bodies.

A strange sensation begins to flow over me, a sensation of intense involvement in, yet also distance from, this event. Perhaps this is what an athlete feels when he has pushed so hard for so long to such a point of exhaustion that all sensation leaves him, and all that remains is the effort itself, effort for its own sake. I cannot shake this feeling, although it is not like me.

When the first bag of suspended cells is ready, I personally carry it to the ICU, where the cells will drip into the patients' veins. Ms. Marotto is first. Outside her room, I review with the nurse the blood samples to be collected and the rate of infusion.

"I need two tiger-tops and three green-tops as the last cells are dripping in," I say, referring to test tubes to be filled with blood. The color-coded tops indicate which lab gets which test tube for testing; tiger-tops go to our molecular biology lab. Some of the samples are for immediate analysis, some to freeze for the future. We have frozen samples from each patient who has ever undergone immunotherapy; if we ever want to run tests on them, we can. We need another complete set of samples five minutes after the drip ends, an hour after, four hours after, then one day, two days, and four days after.

This is finally happening. It is happening.

We walk into Ms. Marotto's room and hang the bag of cells from the infusion pump at her bedside. She looks up at it and smiles. She has been through much worse. In fact, she should feel nothing at all; her central line is already in and she will endure no needle sticks.

"I want a twenty-minute drip," I say.

The nurse adjusts the flow so it will take twenty minutes for the bag to empty.

French Anderson, who has worked for as many years on gene therapy as I have on cancer, is at a conference in Miami, but Mike Polvino, who works in his lab, has come to witness the event. He asks Ms. Marotto, "How does it feel to make history?"

"It's exciting," she answers. "All last year I said this would be the year of my miracle. This is the year everything would go away. I'm just so certain I'm going to get well."

The year of my miracle. She has said this again. Her words pierce.

How I hope she is right. I turn away for a moment, unable to face her in her excitement.

Perhaps this gene therapy really will open up a new world for medicine. Perhaps it will announce the coming of a new age. But I feel no euphoria. If it works I will be euphoric. There will be plenty of time for that. But I understand that this experimental therapy is only that—experimental. In the past we have had some magnificent successes. And we have had more failures.

Ms. Marotto and Mr. Antrim have been informed of this but I do not think they quite comprehend it. They do not want to comprehend it. They want it to work. I comprehend it.

Several others, aware of what is transpiring, hover about, smile at Ms. Marotto, wish her well. The nurse attaches the bag to the central line and turns a toggle switch. The cells begin to drip. It is 8:48 A.M., Tuesday, January 29, 1991.

I stand beside her while the cells are infused in case side effects develop. None do.

So much for history.

Twenty-seven minutes later I repeat the procedure with Mr. Antrim. He suffers no side effects either.

What do I feel? I feel relief—relief to have finally begun. And I feel eager—eager to move forward with this treatment and eager to turn my attention back to the laboratory. I feel what Pasteur wrote: "I am on the verge of mysteries and the veil is getting thinner and thinner."

PART ONE

THE PUZZLE

CHAPTER ONE

Mr. James DeAngelo had severe abdominal pain when I first met him in the summer of 1968, in the emergency room at the veterans' hospital in West Roxbury, Massachusetts. From the first, he intrigued me.

There was nothing wild or bizarre about him, or that hinted at the irrational, yet he wore the wizened and sardonic look of a man who understood the ironies of life, and he had the self-confidence of someone who had had the better of those ironies. I thought his demeanor strange considering his situation; he came to the hospital not only because he had fought in World War II but because he had nowhere else to go. Sixty-three years old with a stubble of beard gone grey, obviously down on his luck, he was sitting there suffering alone, without any family around him, waiting for treatment. I would have expected bitterness or resignation from him rather than this aura of secret triumph, this attitude that seemed to say that he knew things that I did not. But it soon became apparent that Mr. DeAngelo's belief that he had mastered something almost occult was well founded, and he presented a mystery of ultimately enormous dimensions, a mystery that would help send me on a lifelong quest.

His symptoms and physical exam suggested a gallbladder problem. To confirm the diagnosis, I ordered a cholecystogram, a test in which patients swallow dye; the dye concentrates in a healthy gallbladder and not in a diseased one. In his case an X ray revealed no sign of the dye, so surgery to remove the gallbladder was indicated.

This much was routine. Mr. DeAngelo also had a large scar on his abdomen, clearly from surgery, and I asked him about it. He had been to this same hospital before, he said, and with a certain amount of pride, recounted a medical history that made no sense. I assumed he was confused about the facts, so rather than question him further I looked up his chart. It revealed an incredible story.

A dozen years earlier he had undergone surgery for cancer. The surgeon had removed one large tumor but had also found others that he could not remove. He had then closed Mr. DeAngelo's incision, offered him no treatment—there was nothing to be done—and sent him home to die.

But here Mr. DeAngelo was.

At most hospitals doctors would probably have dismissed this incongruity as a mistaken diagnosis, assuming that Mr. DeAngelo's presence proved that he could not have had cancer all those years before. But the West Roxbury Veterans Hospital was an unusual place. True, it had the same dreary architecture and atmosphere of other veterans' hospitals, the same drab government-green paint everywhere, the same chain-link fence surrounding the grounds and striped bathrobes issued to patients, which give it a prison-like feel, and the same patient population of generally poor and lonely middle-aged or elderly men. Many had been treated roughly by life, many were cachectic—emaciated, washed out, and malnourished, often a sign of alcoholism—and most clung with a ferocious dignity to their pride in having fought a war. It was a mark they had left on the world. None of that made West Roxbury unusual. What did was the fact that it, unlike other veterans' hospitals, was the home of some of the very brightest, most aggressive, and most eager to learn—and therefore most alert—young surgical residents in the country.

They came because it was a stop on the training circuit for surgeons at the Peter Bent Brigham Hospital in Boston. "The Brigham," as it is known in the country's medical community, was at the time even more ancient and dingy, and in some ways even more primitive than West Roxbury. It lacked air-conditioning and still had large open wards like a barracks. It was also the single most exciting place in the world for surgeons to train, a place of brilliant men and women. The first organ transplants in the world were performed there. Surgery inside the heart was pioneered there. The field of modern neurosurgery was created there. Kidney dialysis was refined there. All this was done by brilliant people, and the most brilliant of them all was its then chief of surgery, Francis "Franny" Moore.

Franny Moore was authoritative and intimidating. In an extraordinary combination of the roles of basic scientist and clinician, he pioneered the use of radioactive isotopes in measuring the body's chemistry, and created the field of surgical metabolism. This brought modern science to surgery and revolutionized patient care. Already white-haired when I first met him, an almost mythic figure, but still with a barrel chest and a physical presence, he dominated with his voice and his mind. The voice was deep, booming, theatrical without being forced; it demanded not only attention but deference. The mind could simply overpower. He always had something original to offer on rounds; he always seemed to put a twist on the facts that no one else had considered and which was not just provocative but penetrating. When the page operator said, "Call 311," his number, my heart would jump.

I was then a junior resident at the Brigham, under his tutelage, and it thrilled me. I felt a part of all that had gone on there in the past and all that was going to be. Every day its surgeons performed complex operations and handled tertiary referrals, patients whom surgeons at other hospitals did not feel capable of treating. It was heady company to be in and all the residents worked with considerable focus; there were seven of us who started together and we called ourselves "The Magnificent Seven" after the movie. We put in eighteen- or twenty-hour days, sometimes two such days in a row, and felt privileged to do it. Few hospitals still force such hours on their doctors, and this change is a good thing, but then we were young, felt we could go forever, and had the sense we were going to war together. Each of us believed we owed the other our absolutely best performance, and each of us gave it. Anything less would be letting our colleagues, our patients, and ourselves down. Not surprisingly, nothing that was unusual or "interesting"—a pregnant word in both science and medicine—escaped us.

But not all operations require brilliance. A surgical resident also needs training in simple and common operations. For this type of training the Brigham sent its residents for several months a year to the general hospital in Fitchburg, a gritty medium-size mill town northwest of Boston, and to West Roxbury.

I had earlier finished my internship at the Brigham, left for four years to get a Ph.D. in biophysics at Harvard, and had just returned for intense surgical training. While in graduate school, which was only a few subway stops away, I had stayed in close touch with my medical friends but had had little contact with patients. Franny sent me first to West Roxbury to work on simpler cases. This was fine with me. Residents looked forward to their rotation at the veterans' hospital because supervision was looser and they were left relatively alone to make their own decisions on diagnosis and treatment. That freedom was important in what came next, too.

And so it was that Mr. DeAngelo came to my attention.

His chart recounted how, twelve years before, Mr. DeAngelo had walked into the hospital suffering from overall malaise, excessive tiredness and weight loss, and severe abdominal pain. He drank and smoked heavily, consuming three to four fifths of whiskey a week and two packs of cigarettes a day. Reading this, I thought he must have been a hard and troubled man; he seemed less so now. X rays had revealed a large mass in his stomach. An exploratory laparotomy—abdominal surgery—was performed.

According to the chart, the surgeon discovered a life-threatening condition: a fist-size tumor in the patient's stomach, three smaller tumors on his liver, and suspiciously hardened lymph nodes. All of these findings are typical of advanced cancer. The surgeon's operative note stated that biopsies had been sent to the pathologist, who not only confirmed the diagnosis of cancer but added that the disease seemed particularly aggressive and fast-growing. In fact, tumor had already replaced part of the liver.

To alleviate Mr. DeAngelo's pain, the surgeon removed the largest mass along with two-thirds of his stomach, but left the cancers growing in the liver and elsewhere. Resecting them would have greatly increased the risk of killing him on the operating table in return for very little potential benefit. The cancer had spread so far and was advancing so rapidly that removal of more tumors might not have added to his life expectancy at all, while the strain of the additional surgery might have filled what time he had left with more suffering.

On the basis of the diagnosis, Mr. DeAngelo's case seemed hopeless. He should have died within a few months after the operation. But five months later, at a follow-up visit to the hospital, he was very much alive, had gained twenty pounds, and had returned to work.

Now, twelve years later, here he was again.

This did not seem possible. Among the tens of millions of cancer victims since medicine and science joined hands in precise diagnoses, there had been only four documented cases—not four a year in the United States, but four, ever, in the world—of spontaneous and complete remission of stomach cancer. Mr. DeAngelo had experienced a spontaneous and complete remission of stomach cancer.

I went immediately to the pathology report to see if the surgeon had misstated the diagnosis. He hadn't. The pathology report concluded unequivocally that the disease was an aggressive cancer.

This could not be correct. There had to have been a mistake. Or perhaps another surgeon at another hospital had performed aggressive surgery and, amazingly, had succeeded in cutting out all the cancer. I talked again with Mr. DeAngelo.

His voice first hinted at annoyance, then gave way to an ironic collegiality, as if he had decided to take me under his wing and teach me. The doctors had told him he was dying, all right. They told him when they opened him up they had found a lot of cancer and had taken out his stomach. That's what they had said. But he had showed them. He was proud of having shown them. No, he hadn't seen any other doctor back then. No, didn't see any faith healer or chiropractor or out-and-out quack either, though he sure as hell said a few prayers. He just got better. Pretty good trick, huh? Doctors didn't know everything. Right, Doc? There was life in these old bones yet.

I was still certain there had to have been a mistake—a misdiagnosis. I asked the current hospital pathologist to pull out of storage and reexamine the actual slides of the tissue from which the diagnosis had been made. He did, placing the slides under a microscope while I looked on. His diagnosis confirmed the original one: a particularly aggressive cancer.

Now I was deeply puzzled. But another explanation—and surely this had to be it—remained possible: People sometimes live for years with large tumors without having any symptoms, and the cancer might have lost its aggressiveness and remained in his abdomen indolent and slow-growing. This happens rarely but it does happen. By fortunate coincidence the cancer must not have invaded vital areas, and had allowed Mr. DeAngelo to live a normal life.

I was determined to find out if this was the case. We were going to remove Mr. DeAngelo's gallbladder anyway. I intended to explore his abdomen thoroughly.

The operation was one of my first as a junior resident; I would hold the scalpel while the senior resident guided me and protected the patient, and me, from mistakes. As I began, it was instantly apparent that Mr. DeAngelo was missing most of his stomach and had internal scars from that twelve-year-old surgery. Without question he was the same patient from whom the tissue on the diagnostic slides had come.

The operation itself was straightforward. There are operations in which the surgeon can do everything properly and still fail, but removing a gallbladder is not one of them. Still, the blade cuts within a few millimeters, perhaps an eighth of an inch, of major arteries, and there are points of moderate complexity where a mistake could prove lethal. Looking somewhat nervously to the senior resident for his imprimatur at each step, I performed the procedure. Then, after finishing, I began to examine Mr. DeAngelo's abdomen.

I was looking for a slow-growing tumor or for any other signs of cancer. Such signs should have been visible. Visual examination revealed no such signs.

But a surgeon's fingers see more than his or her eyes. My fingers prepared to examine his liver. The liver is delicate, fragile, very unlike the stomach, which has a tough and fibrous surface. The liver is soft, yielding to and rolling under the touch; if one does not take care, one's fingers can puncture it and the patient can bleed uncontrollably. Exposed to the air, the liver's surface dries out and becomes even more fragile, like the skin on chocolate pudding. I slipped my gloves into the abdominal cavity to wet my fingers so they would slide easily around it. Then I pushed my gloved hand, palm up, between his liver and rib cage, pressing my fingers up against the ribs to avoid the liver. Then I turned my palm down and carefully, gently felt the liver.

A tumor is easy to identify by touch; it is tough, dense, unyielding, unlike the texture of normal tissue. It seems alien even. This man had had several large tumors on his liver twelve years earlier.

There was nothing there.

I repeated my exploration, certain my fingers must somehow have skipped over something, some roughness, some alteration in the texture, some nodule. Nothing. Absolutely nothing. I was excited now and explored the intestines rapidly but thoroughly, feeling about for lymph nodes, feeling for some sign, any sign, of cancer, going over the same area twice, asking the senior resident for his opinion and the knowledge of his fingers.

Neither of us could find any evidence of cancer anywhere.

This man had had a virulent and untreatable cancer that should have killed him quickly. He had received no treatment whatsoever for his disease from us or from anyone else. And he had been cured.

I was fascinated. *How?* This man's body had cured cancer. *How?*

I rushed out of the operating room and, still dressed in greens, still encrusted with drying blood, called my wife, Alice. She was a nurse, highly skilled.

"You won't believe what I just saw," I said, and told her.

She understood the significance immediately.

The single most important element of good science is to ask an important question. This was an important question. I hated cancer, hated the alienness of it, hated the way it killed, hated the way it chose its victims. If we could somehow understand how this had happened, if we could somehow understand the mechanism, if we could somehow duplicate the mechanism in other patients . . .

Something began to burn in me, something that has never gone out.

Mr. DeAngelo had received no treatment. His own body had cured his cancer. It was likely that his immune system, which defends the body naturally against disease, had reacted to the cancer and destroyed it.

And I knew of an incident unrelated to Mr. DeAngelo in which another patient's body had also destroyed a violent cancer.

A few years earlier surgeons at the Brigham had transplanted a kidney from a person killed in a car accident. The man who received the kidney soon developed cancer throughout his body. The cancer was traced to the transplanted kidney; the kidney was removed and the metastases—the tumors that had sprung up elsewhere in the body from kidney cancer cells traveling through the bloodstream—disappeared. The patient, like Mr. DeAngelo, had cured himself of cancer.

In this case, however, there was no mystery. We knew, at least in a broad sense, how this patient's body had destroyed the cancer. His immune system had acted exactly as it is supposed to.

The body is engaged in a constant struggle for survival and comes under constant attack from foreign invaders such as viruses and bacteria. The chief fortification against attack is the skin and mucous membranes, but once these fortifications are either breached or evaded, the immune system mobilizes.

When the immune system works perfectly, it recognizes and eliminates any substance that does not belong in the body. If this substance is a living organism, such as bacteria, the immune system kills it; if the substance is not alive, such as the poison from a bee sting, the immune system eliminates it. The body remains healthy and active.

When the immune system does not function properly, disease and death result. The most graphic example of this is AIDS: The initials stand for "acquired immune deficiency syndrome." The AIDS virus does not kill directly; instead, it infects and destroys a particular kind of white blood cell. Without this white cell, the immune system cannot attack foreign substances. This deficiency allows other diseases to advance unchallenged and kill.

The first step in defending the body is to identify targets that must be destroyed. To do this, the body has developed an enormously precise mechanism that allows it to screen virtually every cell and substance in the body and differentiate between that which does and does not belong.

The screening is done by a process similar in principle to fingerprinting. Just as each person has unique fingerprints, which are markings on the surface of the body, each person's cells and other substances of his or her body have unique markings on their surfaces. Foreign, invading substances carry different markings.

Just as police use fingerprints from the surface of a body to identify a suspect, the immune system reads the markings on cells and chemicals within the body to distinguish between that which does belong, or "self," and that which does not belong, or "nonself."

The immune system leaves any substance with self markings alone while it targets and attacks any substance marked as nonself. When the immune system overreacts to a nonself substance, the result is an allergy. When the immune system incorrectly identifies something as nonself which should have been identified as self, the result is an autoimmune disease; in these diseases, which include arthritis and multiple sclerosis, the immune system attacks its own body.

The most common experience with an invasion of foreign material occurs when bacteria penetrate a break in the skin and grow. As the bacteria increase, the infection grows and the immune system recognizes the presence of foreign substances. It reacts by concentrating white blood cells, or leukocytes, at the site of the infection. This concentration of leukocytes makes the whitish, viscous fluid known as pus. In the case of a simple cut, the white blood cells almost always kill the bacteria and the infection subsides.

But just as fingerprints can be smeared or hard to read, making it difficult to identify a suspect, the self and nonself markings can be obscured, making it difficult for the immune system to identify a target. The bolder and clearer the nonself marking is, the stronger the response of the immune system.

The immune system also responds with particular violence to transplanted tissue, which practically rings bells announcing that it is nonself. For this reason, whenever someone gets a transplanted organ, he or she takes drugs to suppress the immune response. Otherwise, the recipient's natural defenses will attack the transplanted organ and destroy it. The immunosuppressive drugs are given continuously after a transplant.

The patient at the Brigham who received the cancerous kidney also received drugs suppressing his immune response. The cancerous cells that spread throughout his body and grew into tumors had not come from him; they had come from the transplanted kidney. They were nonself.

When the kidney was removed and the patient was taken off immunosuppressive drugs, his own immune system quickly identified the cancer cells as foreign, as targets to be killed, and destroyed them. So there was no mystery to this patient's curing himself of the disease.

But if the transplant case was not a mystery, Mr. DeAngelo's case was.

A clear consensus of scientists then believed that the body could not mount an immune response to cancer because cancer cells are one's own. They believed that healthy and cancerous cells carried the same self markings and therefore the immune system could not differentiate between them and could not target cancer cells for destruction.

But there were hints that these scientists were wrong. I knew that people with weakened immune systems were more susceptible to some types of cancer than the general population. I knew that, rare as it was, other documented cases of spontaneous remission of cancer had occurred. And I had just seen in Mr. DeAngelo's abdomen where cancer had been and was no more. I had *felt* it. He had cured himself. Obviously he had experienced something extraordinary. But, assuming his immune system had destroyed his cancer, could the immune system of other people be made to do the same? Did he hold some kind of a key?

Immediately after the operation I began to explore possible clues to what had happened and plan an experiment. Not only white blood cells, but many of the substances that combine to mount an immune response are carried in the bloodstream. I wanted to transfuse Mr. DeAngelo's blood into another cancer victim. I wanted to see if Mr. DeAngelo could be used to cure someone else.

First I scanned records of current patients and found someone in the hospital dying of stomach cancer whose blood type matched Mr. DeAngelo's. The hospital's chief of surgery was Brownell "Brownie" Wheeler, now chief of surgery at the University of Massachusetts. I explained my plans to transfuse Mr. DeAngelo's blood and asked permission to conduct the experiment. He agreed and arranged to have the blood bank staff help me. I then spoke with Mr. DeAngelo, explained that his body had in some way performed a miraculous cure, and asked if he would allow me to transfuse his blood to see if it helped someone else.

He laughed. He had gone through a lot worse without helping anybody. He'd be glad to try and he hoped to hell it worked.

Last, I went to the man dying of stomach cancer. I didn't want to raise his hopes and emphasized that I expected nothing to happen, that this was an incredible long shot. But at least there was no risk. If it didn't work he would be no worse off. He was an elderly man. There was little left of him under his striped bathrobe beyond a scarecrow racked by a rasping cough. He smiled wryly and joked that he had spent his life playing long shots; they had never come in for him yet, and he figured he was due. Damn right he wanted to try it.

Despite the unlikelihood of success, I was excited, arranged the transfusion, and stood by as it was carried out. We were all excited and, despite everything, hopeful.

The long shot failed to come in. The patient showed no improvement whatsoever and within two months died of cancer. In retrospect it was a naive experiment—perhaps even then I knew this—almost embarrassing in its simplicity. But I had to try it.

Meanwhile I looked for clues to what had happened in Mr. DeAngelo. There was one. The original pathologist's report observed that the area around the tumor contained dense infiltrations of lymphocytes and eosinophils. These are two specific kinds of leukocytes, white blood cells. Lymphocytes in particular are the killer cells of the immune system.

In addition, Mr. DeAngelo developed a serious stomach infection from the operation, so serious that ten days after the original operation the surgeon had to reopen the wound. Pus was found throughout the abdomen; the wound was drained, disinfected, and closed, and the patient received heavy doses of antibiotics. The infection disappeared and his recovery was routine and uneventful.

There was no automatic connection between the activity of the immune system and the disappearance of the cancer. Millions of cancer victims get infections while they have the disease and die. There was no reason at all to associate the white blood cells with the cancer. No reason at all. Yet . . .

Mr. DeAngelo recovered quickly from his gallbladder operation and went home the day after he donated his blood for the transfusion. I never saw him again. A few weeks later I was gone myself, my rotation at the veterans' hospital complete. I returned to the Brigham, and to Franny Moore, while in the back of my mind an idea was nagging at me.

CHAPTER TWO

It was not surprising that I found Mr. DeAngelo's case compelling. Practically everything I had done in my life had been focused on solving the kind of puzzle he presented.

While still in high school I laid out a plan for myself that was tightly, perhaps even unhealthily, focused and purposeful: to enter a program at the Johns Hopkins University that combined undergraduate and medical education and yielded an M.D. degree in six years instead of the usual eight, then serve my one year of internship, take a leave of absence to get a Ph.D., and return to finish a surgical residency.

When I told my brother, Jerry, who was eleven years older than I and then studying to become a surgeon, that I planned to go to Hopkins, he warned me not to. He conceded that I had intellectual curiosity but said that curiosity would take me only so far, that I needed discipline, too. Based on his perception of my study habits in high school, he thought I was too lazy to succeed at a school as intense and competitive as Hopkins. He may have been right about my habits in high school, but I intended to change. I did go to Hopkins.

There, learning obsessed me. It also thrilled me. In college I began working in the lab—studying melanoma in hamsters—in addition to my courses. My first scientific paper was about this work and was published during my first year of medical school. The summer before medical school began I put the hamsters in cages, drove them to Minnesota, where my brother was working on a Ph.D. after his M.D., and asked him to finish the experiment for me. I knew I would work hard in medical school and would allow nothing to deflect me even momentarily from pursuing my learning. During the Cuban missile crisis, my friends at Hopkins were gripped with terror over the prospect of a confrontation with the Soviet Union—a confrontation that could conceivably have led to nuclear war. They gathered around the communal television in our eating club to listen to John Kennedy address the nation. I went to the library to study.

During my internship I told Franny Moore of my desire to leave, get a Ph.D., and then return for my residency. He opposed this plan and advised me to get more surgical training before going to graduate school. He also had the power to prevent me from doing so simply by requiring me to reapply to the residency program; admission was so competitive I would not be guaranteed acceptance. I wrote him a letter saying that I was twenty-three years old, that at that age one should follow one's instincts, and my instincts were to learn more science. He agreed to my leave of absence.

The work for my Ph.D. at Harvard consumed me. I was young and even passionate about it, as passionate as any revolutionary or mystic. I loved the night. I think secretly all scientists exalt in working alone, surrounded by the urgent private quiet of the dark. I remember the exhilaration of working through the night in the lab, drinking thick pasty coffee that had been on the burner for hours, walking out into the sunrise, grabbing breakfast at a diner and watching the city come to life. To be doing something no one had ever done, to generate rows and columns of numbers that hinted at a solution to a problem no one had solved—the numbers something I had worked hard for, performed experiments to get, and which could penetrate a mystery—to be alone and out on the edge like that, there was no feeling like it in the world.

And like any passion this was a jealous one. Alice O'Connell was the head nurse in the Brigham emergency room, and I met her on my first assignment there as an intern. It was nighttime and slow. I was sitting with my feet up on a desk reading a surgery text, and she called out, "Hey, come over here. I want to show you something pretty."

She promptly led me outside to look at a moon that filled the sky.

It was the beginning of a complex and volatile five-year courtship. I had never met anyone like her—her combination of vitality, spontaneity, and competence still seems unique—but neither of us started out thinking our relationship had a future.

Alice is a strong woman, very different from me, with traits I lack. She is tremendously comfortable with other people because of her extreme confidence in herself, and far superior to me in social situations. But she was determined *not* to marry a doctor; she disliked doctors' egos and knew that a doctor's hours would mean inattention to family. For my part, when we began seeing each other I could not envision marrying her. Alice was a daily communicant in the Catholic church. I felt that for me to marry someone not Jewish would be a betrayal of my people.

But after that first meeting Alice and I spoke or saw each other every night for weeks. She grew up in Mamaroneck, in a lower-middle-class community of largely Irish Catholics just outside New York City. Her independence and strength showed up early. Of uncles, aunts, brothers, cousins, she is the only member of her family to move away and she did so to attend the Yale–New Haven Hospital School of Nursing. Her interest in research brought her to the Brigham, where, at the age of twenty-one and after working there for only a year, she was put in charge of the emergency ward. For her to get that job, at one of the world's great hospitals, at that age and with so little experience testifies to an extraordinary ability.

I looked forward to speaking with her and interrupted my studying for her. I had never done that before. Although not particularly shy around women, until Alice I had allowed myself time to socialize only on weekend nights. I would often not even call a girl during the week and would wait until Saturday morning or even afternoon—when I was sure I had no work that took precedence—to ask for a date that night.

She was interfering with my life. I wanted to devour knowledge and have nothing interfere. There was almost a ruthlessness to my pursuit. It was unnerving, even unacceptable to me to be involved with someone who could have the kind of impact on me or power over me that she had. It completely disoriented me and I simply stopped calling or seeing her. After ten days of silence she finally called and demanded an explanation. I agreed to meet her at a coffeehouse in Brigham Square. She says that I told her—I don't remember but she insists that she can quote me verbatim—"You're getting in my way. I'm very young, have a lot of work ahead of me, and cannot be distracted. I cannot allow myself to get involved in a relationship that takes my mind off my work. I just can't. We can't see each other anymore. Otherwise it will be too difficult to break it off. It will be too late."

She laughed and said, "It's already too late."

I hesitated, then agreed. "You're right."

She later said that she had gotten my message: that I would not be distracted from my work.

Her description of this meeting, and of me, is chilling. I dislike hearing it. But it rings true. Our problems did not go away. Ultimately my relationship with her distracted me enough from my goal, disturbed me enough that I went briefly to Harvard's psychiatric counseling service. It wasn't easy for her either. Four years later, a year before we married—and before we had talked seriously of marriage—she told me she was converting to Judaism and learning Hebrew. I had not asked her to do this but it marked the intensity of her commitment to me. To her parents, this was anathema. At the same time, we had been seeing each other for four and a half years before I mentioned her existence to my parents. My parents were reluctant to accept her; her family was reluctant to accept me. At our wedding we did not know whether her father would enter the synagogue, although he finally did.

Alice and I met while I was an intern. We married as I finished graduate school. In the interim my education continued.

. . .

To me, education is a process in which one loses one's fear of what one does not know. I knew biologists who were frightened away from a scientific article and stopped reading it when they encountered a differential equation. They were intimidated by their ignorance. I did not want ever to be intimidated by my ignorance. I did not want to be compelled to choose a particular approach to solve a problem at some future date simply because it was the only approach I understood. I wanted to develop confidence that my background was solid enough to allow me to understand anything in science if I made the effort to learn it.

Therefore I wanted to prepare myself in a general way. For example, I was interested in immunology as far back as high school, but rather than study immunology, I studied biophysics.

My course work included advanced calculus, differential equations, electricity and magnetism, thermodynamics, physics, physical chemistry. I hoped this knowledge would allow me to move in any direction, use any tool that seemed likely to solve some future problem. My goal was to understand these subjects at a conceptual level as deep and profound as I was able to grasp, and at the minimum to understand them well enough to be able to learn more about them later if necessary.

At the same time, I studied basic biology. Learning biology, like medicine, required absorbing an enormous volume of facts rather than concepts. Leo Szilard, a prominent physicist who became a biologist, once complained that after he switched to biology he never had a peaceful bath again. Physics is logical; he could sit in his bathtub and think through a problem. Biology is not logical. Every time he tried to get comfortable in the warm water and consider a problem, he had to get up and look up a fact.

Evolution explains the illogic of biology. As life evolves to meet new situations, it cannot choose the best design to meet the situation. It must adjust to what already exists. It must build on what came before. Biology and evolution resemble trying to make an eighteenth-century farmhouse energy-efficient. One has to work with, build upon, add onto, seal and caulk and insulate what already is; the final result will differ radically from a newly built farmhouse designed from scratch to maximize energy efficiency.

When it came time to stop taking courses, combine concepts and facts, and start doing science in the lab full-time, I had to choose with whom to work. Already I had spent one summer doing molecular biology in the lab of Jim Watson and Walter Gilbert. Gilbert would later win a Nobel prize. Watson already had. He and Francis Crick shared it for discovering the structure of DNA, deoxyribonucleic acid. All living cells, whether a single bacterium or each of the trillions of cells in man, contain DNA. DNA is a long, double-threaded and twisted molecule (the DNA from a single human cell would stretch out six feet if unwound). It is the basis of life, and also the nexus between physics and biology. The DNA molecule came into being at such an early stage of evolution that it is more physics than biology. It is so logical as to approach tautology; indeed, it may be the most perfect form in nature.

What struck me most about Watson was that here was a man who had made one of the seminal discoveries of the century yet everyone called him "Jim." Extremely down-to-earth, he carried no airs and did not stand on ceremony at all. The collegiality encouraged creativity and thinking. One had the feeling he would talk to anyone exactly the same way he would talk to Crick. But he also expected people to be like Crick. He expected people to have brilliant insights on their own and to stimulate him. If he thought one's mind worthy of attention, he paid attention; if not, one almost seemed not to exist as far as he was concerned.

Gilbert was a physicist—Crick had also been trained as a physicist—who had been recruited into molecular biology by Watson. He was a difficult man to be around, almost impossible to talk to. Always smoking a pipe, he would bite down on it when asked a question, think for a long moment, take a puff, and reply, "Yes" or "No." One could wait forever for him to elaborate. He was also brilliant and had tremendous and deep scientific intuition.

The attitude of the entire department toward graduate students was simply to drop them in the lab and see who could survive. We were each mainly on our own. And I was generally considered the lowest-ranking member of the department. The reason was simple: In general, basic scientists engage in purely intellectual and, if they are good, creative pursuits, as creative as poetry. They see clinical medicine as mundane and uncreative, and see doctors as glorified plumbers who lack the intellectual ability or creativity to do real science. Everyone knew I not only had an M.D. but intended to return to a surgical residency after graduate school; they viewed me as a strange fish. Watson and his peers were constructing the foundation of a new science, molecular biology, which would reorder the world. Everyone from the secretaries up knew they were making a revolution; the lab vibrated with excitement and intensity.

The excitement did affect me. I never lost sight of my own goal, which was to apply advances made in basic, pure science to patients as rapidly as possible. And I thought that molecular biology was less likely to help solve a clinical problem than many other areas I might pursue for my dissertation. But Gilbert was so impressive I just wanted to be around him and learn. I asked to join his lab and finish my Ph.D. under him.

My decision to ask Gilbert to be my adviser may have been the last time I consciously chose to do something simply because it was intellectually exciting, even though it would divert me from my path. He rejected me. Perhaps he did so because I would be returning to surgery. At any rate, he would not have me. He pushed me back onto my straight-line path. There would be no more diversions.

So I worked with Guido Guidotti and John Edsall—who were brilliant scientists—on protein chemistry. Proteins serve as a crucial element in nearly all tissues—like bricks, they can be used as building blocks of tissue—but they also play crucial roles in most chemical reactions that occur in the body. In addition, proteins serve as messengers carrying information. Every cell in the body makes proteins.

My Ph.D. thesis examined proteins on cell membranes, the surface of the cell that is exposed to the outside world. One role of these particular proteins is to make up the cell surface markings, the fingerprints, which the immune system uses to identify what is self and nonself—to identify what it should leave alone and what it should kill.

And I began to choose a target for myself.

My plan was to build a base of knowledge upon which to stand, and then focus on a specific field. I considered several areas but always seemed to return to cancer. Both the intellectual challenge and my family pulled me toward it. It was not that my parents pushed me toward becoming a doctor or a scientist, nor did they ever push me toward concentrating on cancer. Yet I think that my parents' history and my upbringing were very much at the root of my decision.

My father was born in 1897 in Rajan, a small town in Poland, and had nine brothers and sisters. His father and one brother were killed before his eyes when the family house was shelled by the Germans in World War I. His mother died shortly after with a fever, while he took her in a cart from hospital to hospital, searching for one that would treat a Jew. Soldiers stole his cart. Several times he told me how he cradled her in his arms at the side of the road as she died. On his own, wandering through Europe, he earned enough money to buy passage to America, and he arrived in 1919, twenty-two years old. He worked in a dress factory in New York and as soon as he saved enough money, brought his younger sister and brother to America, where they lived in a small room on the Lower East Side of Manhattan.

My mother was born in 1906 in Michnitz, not far from Rajan. Her father was a merchant with a successful lumber business, but lost everything in the pogroms against the Jews before the First World War. For the duration of the war the family was separated; my mother, her mother, and a younger sister spent much of it hiding in cellars to avoid both the German and Russian armies, and living off the kindness of strangers. They were always hungry. After the war the family was reunited and came to America in 1920. My mother's nine-month-old sister, Rifkah, died a few days after the family arrived at Ellis Island. To pay for the burial of her child, my grandmother sold a string of pearls she had

31

received from her husband as a wedding present. My mother was then fourteen and immediately went to work sewing women's underwear for twelve hours a day and $8 a week. She kept this job until, after a two-year courtship, she married my father in 1927.

By then, my father had become a foreman but life remained hard. My brother, Jerry, was born in 1929. That same year my father lost his job but used all his savings to buy a small candy store in a poor neighborhood on Koskiosko Street in lower Manhattan. Two years later, my sister, Florence, was born and my father traded in the candy store for the first of a series of luncheonettes, which he ran for the next thirty-seven years. I was born in 1940, just after my parents moved to a two-bedroom apartment in the Bronx.

My father was always working. He left the house each morning at 5:30 A.M. to open for breakfast and never returned until after 7:00 P.M. By the time he got home he was exhausted and we never spent much time together. My mother worked in the various luncheonettes and my brother, sister, and I all worked intermittently there after school and during summers. My brother worked at a luncheonette called Donley's, on 23rd Street in Manhattan, which my father owned for fifteen years, and I at the New Madison luncheonette on 32nd Street, which my father bought in 1953. He owned that for fifteen years as well, until 1968. Then, just after Alice and I were married, he and my mother emigrated to Israel. He had always talked and dreamed of living in Israel. My father died there, on September 2, 1991, and my mother now lives alone in Tel Aviv. She wants to live out her life there, refusing our entreaties to return to America, and we each visit her once or twice a year and call her weekly.

My parents' influence on me was profound but subtle. No matter how early I got up in the morning, my father had already left for work. And my own experience in the luncheonette taught me an enormous amount about life, about how difficult it could be—not only my father's but those of his more Runyonesque customers—and about how hard one must work to accomplish anything.

It was not only my father's hard work that influenced me, but my parents' suffering. They never forgot their youth in Poland. And I never forgot the months after World War II, when my parents tried to reach relatives who had stayed in Poland. One after another, my parents sent inquiries about a brother, a cousin, an aunt, a niece. I recall the form postcards that came back from Europe, one after another after another, regretting to inform us that the brother was dead, the cousin, dead, the aunt, dead, the niece, dead, each one murdered in the death camps. I recall the depth of the silence in the apartment with which each postcard was received. Both my father and my mother had gone through something that I could never understand, but I knew what pain was. I wanted to stop their pain, stop everyone's pain. This was not the sole source of my desire to become a doctor but it was a major part of it.

Neither my father nor my mother had much time for education and neither got past the fifth grade. They did not push me to study and did not seem to want me to work too hard. They wanted to make things easy for me. But I always seemed to do well in school without much effort and it was always just assumed I would continue my education.

It was my brother, Jerry, and my sister, Florence, who pushed my education. They inundated me with books on every subject. My sister, who went to work after high school because my parents could not afford to send both her and my brother to college, bought me a new book each payday. We were Orthodox, which meant that on Saturdays we could not turn on electric lights or the radio, talk on the telephone, or travel. I read all day, often on the roof of our apartment building in the summer where the light was better, often finishing in one day whatever book I had just been given. My brother, now a thoracic surgeon in Detroit and a professor of surgery at Wayne State Medical School, also gave me books, usually about science. He was then studying medicine and was my role model. He believed that if he gave me enough stimulation, something would excite me, something would click. He was right.

I read comic books, too, and enjoyed the movies, but I recall my first ambition, aside from becoming a cowboy, was to become a doctor and a scientist. They were heroes to me, exciting; I often cut out newspaper articles about the exploits of a scientist or a doctor, kept them in a scrapbook, and daydreamed about them.

"Doctor" and "scientist" went together in my mind. When I was barely a teenager my brother gave me one particular book I recall about tissue culture, growing animal cells in the laboratory. The challenge of doing this—and the very concept of keeping something alive outside the body—enthralled me. I still have the book.

From my very first interest in medicine as a boy, I wanted to combine research and clinical work. I intended to master medicine and probe deeply into the nature of disease. The goal never varied.

By then of course my brother was often talking about surgery. It was also my brother who pushed me and inspired me, who insisted I study, who insisted my grades were not good enough, who called me lazy. In fact, my mother watched my brother drive himself and because of his obsession objected when I said I, too, wanted to become a doctor. It wasn't worth it, she said. It was too hard. But it was all I wanted.

Indirectly, my family history accounts for my choosing to work on cancer. To me the disease resembles a holocaust. It is a disease one can hate. Other diseases, including heart disease, tend to attack older people, but cancer kills randomly, and it kills the young. Among people between the ages of fifteen and thirty-five cancer kills more than any other disease. In cancer, one's own cells turn alien and grow out of control. Tumors thicken, grow, spread, and eat away at the body. The way cancer gradually takes over one's body and forces its victims and their families to watch impotently as it grows and spreads makes it hateful. Cancer murders innocents. It is a holocaust.

And cancer presents an extraordinary intellectual challenge. The disease represents the central mystery of life, or actually a corruption of that mystery. Exploring this mystery—this was something difficult and profound.

To understand cancer one has to penetrate almost to the very nature of being, to the question of how life develops. All the cells of a life form derive from one cell (in man, this of course is the one cell formed when sperm and egg combine), and contain identical DNA. So each one of the trillions of individual cells in a man or a woman contains the exact same DNA, the exact same genes. Yet somehow each cell grows in a controlled and organized manner, stops growing at a certain point—a finger grows so long but no longer—and differentiates into the heart, the lungs, the hands, the brain.

But how does a cell know when to start or stop growing? How do some cells become a fingernail and others become the heart? These questions of how cells grow and how cells carrying identical genetic information differentiate involve one of the basic puzzles of life, and go to the essence of what we are and how we become it.

In a way, cancer raises this same basic question of cell growth and differentiation. Cancer cells are defined by two traits: They grow at an uncontrolled rate and, unlike other cells, they can grow in, or spread to, different sites of the body.

Cancer *is* uncontrolled, unstoppable growth. Tumors form as cancer cells grow, split, increase in number, and aggregate. Cell presses against cell, increasing the density of cells in cancerous tissue, giving the tumor the dense, hard feel that makes it seem alien and inhuman. When this out-of-control growth presses against or invades nerves, it causes intense, searing pain, which can make cancer the most painful of diseases. Cancer kills when a tumor invades a vital organ or interferes with a vital process.

Cancer also spreads. It metastasizes. Cancer cells are the only cells in the body that can break loose from one site, travel through the bloodstream to another site, and grow. A normal kidney cell will not grow in the lung. But a cancerous kidney cell can lodge in the lung, divide over and over there, growing until the lung is replaced by dense, impenetrable tumor, which blocks the exchange of oxygen and kills.

Cancer is so similar to the normal processes of life that studying it, understanding it has to yield basic knowledge about life itself.

I was particularly curious about a new approach to the disease—an immunological approach. One reason for this curiosity was my experience with Mr. DeAngelo and my knowledge of the earlier Brigham patient who received the transplanted cancerous kidney, and whose immune system destroyed this foreign cancer. But immunology had interested me for many years anyway. My brother had done work in organ transplantation and we had often discussed it. The key to a successful organ transplant is to get the patient's immune system to accept, rather than attack, the foreign organ. Applying immunology to cancer was the exact converse of that problem; the struggle would be to try to get the immune system to recognize a native cancer as foreign and attack it.

I finished graduate school, then returned to the Brigham as a surgical resident. I stayed for only one year and then took another leave of absence to do research in immunology at Harvard. After one year there, in 1970, I joined the Public Health Service and became an immunology fellow at the National Cancer Institute, a part of the National Institutes of Health. It was my first exposure to NIH and it excited me.

In many ways, this experience at NIH was the best time of my life. My first child, Beth, was born. I had the freedom in the lab to pursue any interest, and the resources to support my pursuit. And I had no other responsibilities—no administrative duties, no nights on call in the hospital away from home, no personnel decisions to make, no grant proposals to write seeking money. And surrounding me at the time were some of the finest young minds in the country, largely because of Vietnam.

Doctors interested in research often sought positions at NIH and, if they found them, joined the Public Health Service under the surgeon general of the United States. This government service exempted them from the draft. As a practical result, talented people who might otherwise have pursued research at Memorial Sloan-Kettering Hospital or Stanford University or the University of Michigan or other outstanding institutions congregated instead in the Washington suburb of Bethesda, Maryland, on the campus of NIH. Their brilliance and creativity made NIH an extraordinary place and helped transform it into by far the leading biomedical research facility in the world. The intellectual capital and scientific infrastructure built up during this period—while NIH funding was also exploding—was large enough that the scientific community is still drawing on it.

In the lab I was trying to find tumor antigens. Antigens are part of the identification system that distinguishes self from nonself. I felt I was both learning an enormous amount and making progress in science. The one thing that troubled me was having to abandon my experiments when my fellowship appointment expired. I would have to return to Boston to finish my surgical training. Yet I was now in my thirties, married, and had a child. I had spent seven out of the preceding eight years not in medicine treating patients but in science. To leave science, to return to my residency, to do what people in their mid-twenties did, to be going backwards like that . . . It was tremendously unsettling.

Then Bill Terry, who ran the immunology department at the National Cancer Institute, offered me a senior position. It was tempting. My closest friend, David Sachs, was in the same situation. We had met several years earlier in Boston when he had heard that I, like he, wanted to do research as well as surgery. We talked about our situation over and over. He decided to stay, and never did finish his surgical residency.

But my problem was different. My ambitions were different. I wanted to do something unique. Many people can do research. Many are excellent doctors. Few—very, very few—can both do research and then apply their research to patients. Some try it, but sooner or later almost everyone chooses either the clinic or the lab.

I wanted both. If I was not a clinician and found something that could be applied to patients, I would have to convince a clinician to use my idea. The idea of all my research hanging on someone else's goodwill, of losing control of my work at the moment it is applied to people, did not excite me.

But as a surgeon, I would control the large things—like the design of a clinical protocol—and the small things—like getting access to cancerous tissue for experiments.

I talked to Franny Moore and asked him if there was any way he could get me, as a surgical resident, a laboratory. He agreed, and agreed as well to pay for it and a technician out of his own budget. And so I returned to Boston.

The two years it took to finish my residency were difficult. I was older than everyone else. So was Alice, who expressed the same edge I felt when she joked that she was the only resident's wife in history to have hot flashes. Lying on a cot every other night in the on-call room and staring at a naked light bulb was something for a younger man to do. And my hours were murderous. Up at 5:00 A.M. to read and see patients before going into the O.R. at 7:30, remaining there until 5:00 P.M. or later, then checking on preoperative and postoperative patient care, next doing paperwork or reviewing research, and only then going home at 9:00—if I went home at all.

A surgical residency requires more time than other specialties, and it has always had a macho mythos. Typical of this mythos, when someone asked one of my colleagues if he disliked working every other night, he said, "Yeah. You miss half the cases."

But the reality was brutal, especially for someone in his thirties with a family. The sleep deprivation was killing. I routinely fell asleep at red lights on the drive home. Once another resident and I both fell asleep at a patient's bedside. I swore that if ever I controlled residents' schedules I would not put them through this. After a resident's fatigue contributed to the well-publicized death of one patient in New York, several states passed laws limiting the hours residents work.

My lab, one small room, was across the street from the Brigham at the Harvard Medical School. Alan Baker, who had also been a fellow at NIH and had just finished his residency at the Brigham, worked with me in the lab for six months. My technician was Susan Schwarz. My scientific progress in this lab was limited at best, but this marked the beginning of a relationship with both people that has continued unbroken for twenty years.

Sue and I actually met face-to-face only once a week or so, but she would write down the results of her experiments, and early in the morning or late at night I would review them and write her instructions about what experiments to do next.

In the lab and in my residency my focus was on cancer. I wanted to learn the disease, learn it as well as possible at the molecular level and at the level of basic science, learn everything about its clinical manifestations, learn everything about treatments for it. It was my enemy, and I wanted to know my enemy and grow intimate with it.

Whenever possible, I went to oncology conferences to learn about chemotherapy, and I also exchanged my rotation in cardiac surgery for one in radiation therapy. This was highly unusual. As a surgical resident, in theory I was to work only in surgery. But Franny let me go. It was one more indication of his graciousness and approval.

Finally the two years ended. Finally my formal training was finished. I had spent my entire life in training. College, medical school, internship, graduate school, residency, two fellowships, more residency. It was time, finally, to move forward.

By then the "War on Cancer" was just reaching full speed and hundreds of millions, ultimately billions, of dollars were being directed toward cancer research. In Washington, advocates for what have become known as "disease constituencies" play exactly the same role as lobbyists for other constituencies. The anticancer crusade was created by activists—particularly Mary Lasker, a wealthy philanthropist who had been friendly with politicians for decades, and the American Cancer Society—and by presidential politics.

These activists claimed a precedent for their crusade: In 1961 John F. Kennedy had set a goal of landing a man on the moon by the end of the decade. In December 1969, just a few months after the moon landing, Lasker and her allies launched their effort publicly with a full-page ad in *The New York Times* headlined, MR. NIXON: YOU CAN CURE CANCER.

The ad quoted Dr. Sidney Farber, a prominent Harvard cancer researcher who was also a golf partner of former President Dwight Eisenhower, saying that a cure was close at hand and lacked only money, will, and an organized program to bring it to fruition. The crusaders demanded that a new national goal be set: Cure cancer by 1976 to celebrate the nation's two-hundredth birthday. Despite Vietnam, the nation still had enormous self-confidence and technologically all things still seemed possible—including this goal.

The Nixon administration initially resisted the call for a war on cancer, but the 1970 election changed the political equation. Senator Ralph Yarborough, a liberal Texas Democrat, was defeated in the primary by Lloyd Bentsen, who then defeated George Bush in the general election.

Yarborough had chaired the subcommittee that funded NIH. His replacement as chairman was Senator Edward Kennedy, a potential rival of Nixon's for the presidency. (Two years later Kennedy's son would lose a leg to cancer.)

Suddenly Nixon reversed himself. In his January 1971 State of the Union message, he jumped on the cancer crusade bandwagon. In December 1971 he signed the National Cancer Act.

The law flooded cancer research with money and even allowed the head of NCI to take his budget request directly to the president, over the heads of his nominal superiors. This was unlike any other reporting arrangement in the federal government.

Unfortunately, the idea of capping the 1976 bicentennial celebration by curing cancer was naive, even absurd. The problems of cancer and getting to the moon had little in common.

Putting a man on the moon was a tremendous engineering feat, but it was mainly engineering. When John Kennedy set the goal, American engineers already knew the physics, the mathematics, the basic knowledge of the structure of metals necessary to succeed. No new scientific principles had to be developed.

Curing cancer was a different task entirely. Although we had made some progress at that point in treating the disease, we lacked the kind of deep understanding necessary to find a cure. We did not know enough even to know where to look for one.

The War on Cancer provided my first view of the politics of science, and it came from afar. It would not be my last, and other encounters would come at a distance close enough to call intimate.

But if this war was oversold to the public and to Congress, and if it was being waged as part of the political tug-of-war of presidential politics, the result was that enormous amounts of energy and money poured into research efforts. It was in this context, about eighteen months after the signing of the National Cancer Act, that I began looking for my first real job.

CHAPTER THREE

Franny Moore wanted me to stay in Boston. He offered me the job of chief of surgery at Harvard's brand-new Dana/Farber Cancer Center, which would be directly across the street from the Brigham in a seventeen-story building then under construction.

This was obviously a tremendous offer. The job would carry with it the rank of professor at Harvard, give me the chance to set up an entire program from scratch, and allow me to maintain my association with the Brigham, with Harvard, with the entire medical and research community of Boston. It also carried enormous prestige. In theory, at least, I would become Franny's peer. For someone just finishing his residency, who was not yet even a board-certified surgeon (a surgeon has to finish residency before being allowed to take the boards), this was a tremendous offer indeed.

Yet I was not entirely enthusiastic about it. Organizing a completely new unit at a place as political and turf-conscious as Harvard Medical School would be difficult, and it quickly became apparent that I would be waging a war over turf. Except for Franny, the entire Boston scene with which I would be interacting seemed jealous and competitive. There was more rivalry between research groups than I thought healthy, and too often clinicians and researchers had little intercourse. And in my struggles I would be at a disadvantage. Practically everyone I would have to fight with was already a Harvard full professor with an existing network of bureaucratic, medical, and scientific allies. Although by then I had published more than thirty scientific papers, I was still only a resident who was supposed to become their equal overnight.

Before agreeing to the Dana/Farber offer, I visited NIH and sat down with Nat Berlin, the National Cancer Institute's scientific director; Bill Terry, who ran NCI's immunology branch and had earlier offered me a research position there; and Alfred Ketcham, chief of the NCI Surgery Branch, to see if we could work out something suitable for me there.

Alf Ketcham was a big, bold man who believed in ever bigger and ever bolder operations. Alf was dynamic, gruff, gregarious, and outgoing—a swashbuckling prototype of a surgeon, charging through doors, issuing orders, snapping out jokes. He lived in the O.R., loved to be with patients. Under him the Surgery Branch was a macho place; on every desk was a sign with the letters YCCCSOYA, which stood for "You Can't Cure Cancer Sitting On Your Ass."

I think Alf viewed his role as advancing surgical techniques, learning how to do larger and more complex operations, and training residents and visiting fellows in these techniques. He wanted NCI to become the world center for huge, difficult operations.

My view of what the branch should have been doing differed radically from his. As aggressive as the Surgery Branch was under Alf, little serious laboratory research was being conducted, and dozens of teaching hospitals around the country could do and were doing what he was doing. Yet NCI had a mixture of laboratory and clinical resources that could not be duplicated anywhere else in the world. I believed NCI should do only those things that no one else could.

My conception of surgery also differed radically from Alf's. I love to perform surgery but consider it one of many tools, and one with obvious limits; too often cancer is inoperable, and too often it recurs after surgery. And the problem with the huge operations Alf was performing was the one single cancer cell that escaped his knife, found a home in another part of the body, and grew. On the wall behind my desk is a quote that would make Alf recoil in pain. John Hunter, the famous eighteenth-century surgeon who helped transform medicine into a science, said, "Surgery is like an armed savage who attempts to get that by force which a civilized man would get by stratagem."

Perhaps not surprisingly, Alf wouldn't allow me the independence I wanted or sufficient time to do research. We could not work out a mutually satisfactory position for me to fill.

I returned to Boston and accepted the Dana/Farber position.

Even so, I made my acceptance conditional on certain needs being met and detailed them in a long letter to Tom Frei, who had been hired as physician-in-chief of the center from M. D. Anderson Hospital in Houston and who before that had headed the Medicine Branch at the National Cancer Institute. We began negotiations.

One point of contention between Frei and myself epitomized the turf war that could soon engulf me. This new cancer center was being designed without an operating room. The center was to use the O.R. at the Brigham. Patients would be wheeled from one building to the other through a tunnel.

I was reluctant to accept this situation—to be a chief of surgery without an operating room. Any chief of surgery has to control the operating schedule and, particularly in a research setting, has to be able to set his or her own priorities. Instead of supporting my request that the center have its own O.R., Frei fought me over it. He and I went round and round on this point.

Meanwhile things were about to change abruptly at NCI. Alf Ketcham had been there for years, and stratagem was more in keeping with the new War on Cancer—with its emphasis on research, with the power and money that flooded into NCI—than was Alf's approach of blazing six-guns. Tension developed between him and those who wanted to push the Surgery Branch toward the lab.

Alf had six children and they were approaching college age. Regardless of his attitude toward laboratory research, he was an outstanding clinical surgeon. He regularly received job offers at literally triple and quadruple his government salary.

After I had tentatively accepted the Dana/Farber position and while I was negotiating several items, Alf Ketcham announced his plans to leave NCI. Nat Berlin, NCI's scientific director, began looking for a replacement.

When Ketcham announced that he was leaving, Bill Terry urged Berlin to offer me the job. Initially Berlin resisted for the obvious reason: How could he consider offering someone who was just finishing his clinical training a position as chief of surgery?

But Nat is an interesting man. If he decided to do something, it got done. Short and thin, diminutive in every physical way, he still had, and has, a commanding presence. And his post as scientific director gave him real power inside NIH. Nat recalls, "In those days [we] scientific directors of the various institutes . . . called ourselves the College of Cardinals and used to meet twice a month. We held in our hands space, positions, and budget for each research unit. We were very supportive of one another. Individually and collectively we were a very influential group."

I believe the fact that I had been offered the Dana/Farber position made him take me seriously as a candidate. That was the strongest endorsement possible from Franny Moore. And Bill Terry continued to push my name.

Meanwhile the chiefs of several clinical services met with him and asked that he appoint a search committee. He received this idea with even less warmth than Terry's suggestion. Finding someone was his responsibility—and within his power—and he was not about to yield any authority. As he later recounted, he went around the table and asked each of them how they got their jobs. "You appointed me, Nat," was the universal answer. Then they thanked him for seeing them.

There was no search committee, but Nat did set up two advisory groups of highly respected surgeons, including Franny Moore, and asked for advice about the background the next chief of surgery should have, and the directions in which the surgical branch should proceed. Both groups recommended that he find someone with a strong research background. Bill Terry persisted, mentioning me again.

Berlin felt Franny out about me and ran into resistance—I had already accepted the Dana/Farber position—which made Berlin more interested than ever. Franny suggested he talk with a friend of mine, Paul Sugarbaker, about the job but Berlin did not. Instead he asked Franny's permission to interview me and got it.

I knew I wanted the NIH job. Hospitals and universities could pay a good surgeon much more than what NIH paid. But the government certainly paid enough to raise a family, and one doesn't miss money if one has never had it. Alice and I had never had it. And Alice was content to do—in fact she was intent on doing—whatever was best for my work rather than pressuring me to increase my income. We had enough to have bought a small house in Wellesley, ten miles from Boston, where our second daughter, Rachel, was born the previous year. We felt we had enough.

But if NIH paid lower salaries, it poured money into other areas. It had everything—absolutely everything—I wanted. No university or hospital in the world could match its resources, its depth of scientific knowledge, its laboratory space, its research beds, and its deep pockets. At every other hospital, researchers war constantly with hospital administrators over who pays the several-hundred-dollars-a-day charge for a hospital bed; most health insurance programs will not pay for experimental treatments. At NIH the government pays. To take an idea from the lab directly to clinical trials, there was simply no place like it.

Equally important, at NIH scientists are free to do science. They do not worry about funding. In the academic world scientists have to spend an inordinate amount of time, often one-quarter and sometimes up to one-third of their time, writing grant proposals to pay for their research. In fact, much of this research money comes from NIH itself.

Berlin came up to Boston and we met in Franny's library. The meeting was informal but it could not be termed casual. I had prepared for hours, organizing and rehearsing what to say about the research I thought could be done at the branch. Berlin, a scientist, was receptive.

A few weeks later my beeper went off in C-Main, a huge open

46

ward. I picked up the phone. It was Berlin. "I want to offer you the job," he said.

All I had ever wanted to do in my life was medical research, and to apply what I found directly to patients. No place in the world could compete with NIH for the chance to do that. I knew I wanted the job but couldn't say yes then—I had to talk to Franny first. He had to hear it from me.

Berlin said, "Okay, but before you settle on anything else be sure to get back to me."

I called Alice. She knew what Harvard was like and knew we had had two wonderful years at NIH. Her immediate reply was, "I'll start packing."

Then I called Franny and told him I had to come see him right away. It was the most difficult moment of our long relationship. I had not signed anything on the Dana/Farber offer, had always made clear that my acceptance was contingent upon certain conditions being met, and we were not making much progress toward meeting those conditions. But I had accepted. Now I was going to his office to back out.

His office was dominated by a huge desk but had the feel of a den. In front of a large window there were two easy chairs at an angle, turned half toward the window and half toward each other. He gestured for me to take one and sat in the other.

"I'm changing my mind," I blurted out. "Berlin offered me the NCI job. I'm going to take it."

He listened for a moment, pensively looking out the window, then with the full weight of his authority said, "I think you'd be making a mistake to turn the Dana/Farber position down."

If the words were gentle the authority behind them was not. Franny had done extraordinary things for me, and he had done them repeatedly. There was literally no one in the world I respected more than him. I believe he respected me. We did not have a father-son relationship. Franny was always a distant figure, revered rather than loved. But in some ways respect goes deeper than love. I know I am focused. Perhaps focus is another word for ruthlessness. If so, I was ruthless that day. We talked for well over an hour in his office, moving in circles. I tried to leave, even rose to leave, but he insisted and I sat down again, then rose again. He promised me resources and I knew he would keep his promises. But no place had the resources of NIH. I knew I was going there but wanted desperately to convince him NIH would be a better place for me. I could not. As I left he turned away from me, turned toward his desk, leaving me facing his back.

CHAPTER FOUR

The job marked an extraordinary change for me.

On June 30, 1974, I was a senior resident who spent every other night on call in the Brigham, sleeping in a room smaller than some closets, with a naked light bulb hanging from the ceiling, and taking orders from the chief resident and every staff surgeon in the hospital. I had never been in charge in the operating room, never been the most senior surgeon at the table. On July 1, I became chief of surgery at the National Cancer Institute, the largest clinical unit at the National Institutes of Health, controlled an annual budget of millions of dollars, had four secretaries and an administrative assistant, and supervised a dozen prominent senior surgeons, more residents and fellows, and a total staff approaching 100 people.

Some people at NCI were receptive to me. Others were not. One of the nurses told me later—years later—that people referred to me as "the boy wonder," with the emphasis on "boy" and an ironic if not sarcastic inflection on "wonder."

I was not a boy. I was thirty-four years old with two children and frankly frustrated over the delay in beginning what would become my life's work. Every colleague who had started training with me so many years before had long since begun his professional life. I had not. True, they had all mainly pursued clinical surgery, but the knowledge that I had chosen another, longer track did little to ease my frustration at not having proceeded further down it.

Even now I could not simply pursue my own research, which

was my whole purpose in coming to NCI. My first priority had to be administrative; I had to redirect the efforts of other doctors in the branch, and if necessary replace them. My own lab work was put on hold, even to the point that Sue Schwarz, my lab technician in Boston whom I had persuaded to follow me to Bethesda, went to work for my friend Dave Sachs, the immunologist, for six months.

Inevitably there were clashes. The first came over my reorganization of the operating schedule to allow time for research. Previously the surgeons had each had a specialty and had operated whenever a case involving their field of interest came up. This kept them in the O.R. year-round and made it impossible to do excellent research. I created a rotation that put one or two surgeons on the clinical service two to four months a year, and they operated not only on their specialty but on all cases (exceptions were made for particularly complex operations). This gave everyone at least eight uninterrupted months for laboratory research. I began holding two research seminars a week in which doctors told each other what they were doing in the lab.

Some doctors chose to leave. Others were squeezed out. At the research presentation of one senior surgeon, he declared, "I don't like to work with anything I can't see." His research reflected this attitude; he was producing little worthwhile and I reduced his lab space and reassigned his technician to someone who was more productive. I did the same with others whose lab work was poor. Many of these people were excellent technical and teaching surgeons, much more experienced than I in performing complex operations. But none were exceptional scientists, and none were exploiting the unique opportunities NIH offered of applying scientific research directly and immediately to patient care.

Not surprisingly resentment developed and one or two of my colleagues were gunning for me. Some thought that maybe I was a hotshot in the lab—maybe—but wondered if I knew anything about surgery.

The very first case I worked on became much more of a test than it should have been. I assisted Harry Sears, a senior surgeon, in an exploratory laparotomy on a twenty-four-year-old woman with ovarian cancer. She had a virgin belly, one never operated on before. Sears removed a small ovarian tumor and took numerous biopsies. Everything seemed fine and I left. But postoperatively she began to bleed into her belly. It became distended and she required six units of blood. Almost always this means that a tie on a major artery has come off, an uncommon event but a straightforward one to correct.

Sears called me at home. Alice and I were about to go out to dinner. I thought it would take an hour in the operating room to solve the problem—Sears would not need me for the entire operation—and Alice came in with me and waited in my office.

We began routinely. Suddenly the anesthesiologist, his voice panicky, warned, "I'm losing blood pressure and don't know why."

I looked over the drapes. The girl's face was as bloated as a balloon. I pressed her chest and felt air crackling.

It was instantly apparent what had happened. Preoperatively a resident had put in a central catheter and had nicked the lung, creating a pneumothorax. Air was escaping from her lung into surrounding tissue. The routine X rays had been taken after the procedure to check for this, but the pneumothorax had not shown up. Now, with her anesthetized and intubated, a machine was driving air under pressure into her lungs. The tiny seepage of air had become pressurized bursts, forcing air into the soft tissues, distorting them, pushing one whole side of the chest against the other side until the tissue pressed against the blood vessels into the heart—and against the heart itself.

The pressure had to be released.

Immediately I jabbed a large bore needle into the chest wall. Air whooshed out. But the anesthesiologist exclaimed, "The heart just stopped!"

No one can describe the horror of someone dying on the operating table. This was a twenty-four-year-old woman with an entire life to be lived.

She was dead.

I ripped off the drapes covering her body and, not waiting for any sterile prep, slashed an eight-inch-long incision in her chest, put in a rib spreader, and opened the chest cavity, then thrust my hand in. As soon as I felt her heart I began to squeeze it rhythmically, trying to pump blood through her body with my hand.

Simultaneously we needed to increase her volume to raise her blood pressure. We began pouring blood into all her IVs. Then I asked Sears to massage the heart while I cut down on another vein to start another IV—now we had four going, and we were pouring blood into each.

When the volume finally returned, we shocked the heart.

It started.

Ninety minutes into the operation the patient stabilized. Meanwhile we put in a chest tube under suction; it expanded the lung against the chest wall, sealing the original leak and allowing the lung to heal itself. Three hours into the operation we found the bleeder and tied it off.

At 2:00 A.M. I found Alice asleep in my office. I woke her and we went home. Later the patient walked out of the hospital healthy; she did not even have an infection from the lack of a sterile prep for her chest incision.

This was the kind of crisis I had spent the previous two years resolving as a senior resident, operating five to ten hours a day. In reality it was easier for me than some of the operations other surgeons in the branch routinely performed. But it was important. Even if I still lacked the specific technical skill to perform particular operations, such skills can be readily developed if one knows basic techniques. Judgment is harder to develop. This operation showed people in the O.R. that if there was a problem, I could handle it. They began to trust my judgment.

I began learning how to perform the operations the others had been doing. Paul Chretien had been Ketcham's deputy but was passed over as his replacement when I was hired. Yet he was gracious in teaching me and some other surgeon/scientists whom I recruited. He was very shy, very quiet, much my senior, but always wanted to assist me, even when I said, "Paul, I want to see how you do this." Perhaps that was his way of controlling the operation. The first assistant can guide events in some ways better than the chief surgeon. Exposure of the operative field is very important, and if the first assistant produces excellent exposure of tissue, something that could be difficult becomes easy. I owed Paul. I did cut back on his lab resources but made it plain that he could stay as long as he liked.

Meanwhile I began to redefine both the goals of the Surgery Branch and my own life, and established a routine that I have followed ever since.

In my personal life, it was clear that the hospital and the laboratory could easily consume every waking minute and I was determined not to allow that. My father had never been home in time for dinner. I made it a rule always to be home for dinner. I might come into work very early in the morning and return after dinner, but my family and I had dinner together. We bought a house a few minutes from NIH, close enough that travel time would never deter me from returning in the evening.

Alice asked me to keep her informed about my work. I promised to do that; we often took long walks around the block while I tried to explain things to her. I soon found these talks forced me to focus on scientific issues in ways that helped clarify them in my own mind.

Although I went into the hospital on both Saturdays and Sundays, Sunday nights Alice and I went to the movies. This was my one real escape from work. I did not want great art. I did not want to watch a sad movie. I got upset when I saw blood or violence on the screen and often walked out of movies. I also cried easily, so easily that my children were often embarrassed. The tears were part of the escape; in the hospital, professionalism often precludes showing emotion.

At the hospital, in order to guarantee uninterrupted time to concentrate on my own projects, the secretaries were told not to disturb me with nonemergency telephone calls until after 3:00 P.M. Then I would return them. Similarly, I let administrative details pile up each week until Saturday and then dealt with them—at least those not already handled by my administrative assistant, Jeannie Gianini, who had done the same job for

Ketcham and who knew her way around the bureaucracy. Her ability soon became apparent and I relied on her more and more. She is smart and resourceful, and soon handled all my dealings with the federal bureaucracy. I learned that it was not necessary for me to know how something worked. I simply asked Jeannie to take care of it—from finding a way to hire someone who did not quite fit a job description to getting construction work done promptly—and she found a way. Jeannie and her assistant, Joan Chapman, have worked with me all of my years at NIH.

And despite the conflicts that ensued over my efforts to reshape the Surgery Branch into a place of science, I tried to create a collegial and teamlike atmosphere. Oddly enough, my two formal efforts to do this failed.

First came my attempt to change the feel of the place. Most doctors, and especially surgeons, believe in a hierarchy. The O.R. is no place for playing devil's advocate. But hierarchy and authority are anathema to science and the creative process. Impressed by my memory of everyone calling Jim Watson by his first name, I wanted everyone to call me Steve. My brother was appalled by this; he felt that in light of my age I needed to establish authority. But few people did call me by my first name. Over time, I gave up the attempt to get people to do so.

Second, I organized a Surgery Branch basketball team. I have always loved basketball. We had one doctor who had played for Duke, and it seemed to me that a team built around him would be unstoppable. Although the closest to organized basketball I ever got was an after-school recreational league in junior high school, I played point guard for our team. But NIH is a huge place; thousands of people work there. Our first game was against the elevator operators. We lost 116–32. Our second game was against the laundry. All we knew about them was that they had taken the elevator operators apart. It was 30–0 before we got the ball past half-court. I decided basketball at this level wasn't for me. The team continued but I did not.

More to the point, we set up prospective clinical research protocols. Previously, the branch had not run a single one; it had never set up an organized study to answer a question about the effectiveness of a specific treatment. Instead, the branch had treated any patient whose case looked interesting. I reversed this policy. We would accept only cases that answered a question about disease. NCI paid all patient expenses, including travel. The Surgery Branch had not been using the money budgeted for patient travel before; I knew I would and asked that it be expanded.

To ensure objectivity I insisted that patients in many of our protocols have their treatment randomly selected. Prospective randomization can raise hackles in medicine. To run a prospective randomized study a doctor must say to a patient, "We have several treatments that may work equally, but we're not sure which one is best. To find out I'll pick your treatment by a randomized procedure similar to flipping a coin. Is that okay with you?"

Randomized protocols were not new, but they were infrequently used. In the 1700s, James Lind performed one of the first such studies. The British Navy was then plagued by scurvy; on a sea voyage Lind took twelve sailors, divided them into six groups of two each, and gave each group something different to eat. Ten sailors got scurvy. The two who ate limes did not. Hence the British became known as "limeys," and scurvy disappeared from their navy.

Some doctors, including many whom I respect immensely, believe a doctor should always choose the treatment, based on the doctor's best judgment and knowledge of the particular patient. They argue that retrospective studies—studies that look backward into case histories—can supply the data needed to judge the effectiveness of a given therapy, and also claim that patients will not accept a prospective randomized protocol.

I think the truth is that many doctors won't accept randomization. It changes the relationship with the patient and strips away the doctor's authority. Too many doctors are comfortable dealing with patients only when they can assume an air of unquestioned authority. Surgeons tend to be particularly authoritative. I am equally certain that retrospective studies cannot establish most clinical facts; our own clinical research would soon demonstrate this by contradicting some retrospective studies that I had considered convincing.

The Surgery Branch soon began randomized protocols, including several grueling ones on sarcoma that directly involved me.

By then I had been chief of the Surgery Branch for eight months, and had already recruited two of the Brigham's best young surgeons, Al Baker and Paul Sugarbaker, whom Franny had suggested to Nat Berlin for the job as chief. I had convinced them that the opportunities at NIH were unparalleled. Murray Brennan, an outstanding thinker who is now chief of surgery at Memorial Sloan-Kettering Hospital in New York, would soon be coming as well. The branch was beginning to resemble my image of what it should be like. It was time to get back to my own work.

Shortly after taking the NCI job I systematically and exhaustively reviewed the scientific literature on approaches to cancer. My goal was to find, based on what we knew then, the approach that was most likely to work—if we could just *do* it.

There were three avenues to consider: doing basic scientific research in the hope that it would yield something unexpected that would have immediate application; looking for marginal improvements in existing therapies and techniques; or exploring new approaches that my intuition told me might work.

Basic science involved studying the disease mechanism itself. Advances in basic research come in unpredictable ways and at unpredictable times; one follows wherever one's work leads. As Homer Adkins, an organic chemist, once observed, "Basic science is like shooting an arrow into the air and wherever it lands painting the target."

Although basic research is valuable, I did not consider it a viable option for me to pursue. The second option, that of marginally improving existing therapies, also did not attract me. Surgery and radiation therapy were obviously confined to treating local occurrences of the disease. I believed in aggressively using surgery even on metastatic cancer—cancer that has already begun to spread—and I worked extensively in this area. But I also recognized that if a single cancer cell escapes the surgeon's knife, the cancer can recur.

So the real answer to cancer had to be in some systemic treatment of the disease. Chemotherapy, which grew out of World War II research on chemical warfare, treats the disease systemically and real successes were being achieved with it. Already scientists and clinicians had developed drugs and drug combinations that cured leukemias and lymphomas that had been lethal, and chemotherapy would soon be curing 90 percent of cases of testicular cancer that had previously been considered terminal. Gratifying progress was being made.

But there was often little scientific rationale behind many of the investigations of drugs. No one really understood enough about the difference between cancerous and normal cells to know why a drug worked, or to rationally design a drug to affect cancer. I was skeptical that many such drugs existed in nature.

And, the biggest problem with chemotherapy was distinguishing between diseased and healthy tissue. It was easy enough to find a drug that killed cancer cells; it was difficult to find a drug that killed cancer cells but left normal cells untouched. The body already has an incredibly sophisticated device to distinguish between normal cells and deadly threats. It was called the immune system. Why not try to use it?

It is every immunologist's dream to use the immune system to cure cancer. It is every immunologist's nightmare that there is no such thing as an immune response to cancer in humans. At the time of my arrival at NCI, the prevailing view of those scientists investigating both cancer and immunology embraced the nightmare.

One statement of this view appeared in an article in the *British Journal of Cancer* at about the time I moved to NCI. It concluded that no immune response had ever been shown to occur in reaction to a spontaneously arising cancer in animals or man.

The article touched a raw nerve among the small field of tumor immunologists and provoked angry rebuttals from them. It also stirred their deepest fears—that all their efforts were doomed to failure. Tumor immunologists were well aware that not a single clinical experiment had ever succeeded in stimulating an immune response in man that caused a tumor to disappear. Many such experiments had been tried. That was precisely why the field of tumor immunology was so small. Most immunologists, convinced the work would come to nothing, had no intention of wasting their lives on what they considered a fool's errand.

My own feelings were different.

I believed the human immune system could respond to cancer. I was not alone in this belief, but it was held by a distinct minority of scientists. Several pieces of evidence led to this conclusion.

For one thing, it was known that people whose immune systems were in some way suppressed had higher rates of some cancers than the general population. This suggested that a properly functioning immune system could, at least in some cases, prevent cancer from ever developing.

Also, excellent science was being done by a small number of investigators in the field, particularly Alexander Fefer, Karl and Ingegard Hellstrom, George Klein, Richard Prehn, and others. I believed that they had demonstrated that an immune response to cancer could be stimulated in animals. Granted, they had not so much uncovered an immune response as induced, almost forced, one. But they had established that animal immune systems could respond to cancer.

It seemed to me that if something as fundamental as an immune response existed in animals, it should exist in man.

It further seemed to me that, on the basis of all my intuition as well as a systematic review of the scientific literature, the approach that was most likely to work—if we could just *do* it—was one involving the immune system.

And now I had the power to devote significant resources to making this possibility real.

.   .   .

Immunotherapy already had a long history. In the late 1800s two German scientists independently injected cancer patients with cultured streptococci bacteria and claimed benefits, but the best-known experience was in New York. There, William Coley, a surgeon at what is now Memorial Sloan-Kettering Hospital, tried a similar approach and also claimed some success; in fact his treatments became known as "Coley's toxins" but were abandoned when others could not reproduce his findings. The hope was that the bacterial infection excited the immune system enough in a general way that it also attacked the cancer. Coley's daughter set up a foundation to fund research that attempted to prove her father's thesis. A scientist I respect, Lloyd Old, believes Coley's toxins worked and has speculated that they did so by stimulating the production of tumor necrosis factor—a protein that has since played a major role in our own genetic work.

Several scientists, including Donald Morton, who left NCI for UCLA shortly before my arrival, were experimenting with the same concept. They were infecting cancer patients with BCG, a bacterium related to the tuberculosis bacillus. Morton had conducted a retrospective study, comparing survival rates of patients given BCG to the medical histories of other patients, and claimed significant results.

I saw little real intellectual rationale behind this BCG work—no animal data supported the thesis, and the immune system is highly specific; a response to one stimulus, the BCG, should not stimulate a response to another stimulus, cancer. Still, I considered it promising and instituted a prospective randomized protocol to test its effectiveness in patients with bone cancer and melanoma. (This protocol subsequently demonstrated that BCG had no effect on these cancers, but it could put patients through new agonies.)

I did not want to take this blunt and empirical approach. I wanted to develop a hypothesis, probe more deeply into the workings of the immune system, and exploit the great advantage it offered: its precise specificity in attacking foreign invaders. And I thought I had a clue as to how to do this.

I thought T lymphocytes might be the answer.

The basic functioning of the immune system—to identify and distinguish between self and nonself substances in the body and then to eliminate nonself substances—relies upon a complex system of markings on all substances inside the body.

The markings themselves jut out like jagged keys from the surface of, for example, bacteria or foreign cells. Elements of the immune system hold matching locks, which also jut out from their surfaces. Sooner or later in the body, the lock will come into physical contact with the key. If the key fits the lock, a physical bond is formed, identification as nonself is made, and the immune response begins. An immune response always requires this physical binding.

The keys—the markers of nonself substances—are called antigens, which are defined very simply as anything that will stimulate a response from the immune system. Antigens are proteins on cell surfaces.

The locks are called receptors. A receptor binds to an antigen.

Not all receptors are attached to immune system cells. Some circulate in body fluids; these are called antibodies.

Antibodies do not kill. Usually their binding simply marks and targets a substance for destruction by other immune system elements. But antibodies can sometimes neutralize a threat by themselves; they do so by binding to the antigen, which can have the same effect as handcuffing a violent criminal.

At the time I came to NCI and for several decades before that, immunologists were devoting most of their attention to studying antibodies.

There were several reasons for this. Most immune responses, including those to bacterial infections, involve antibodies, and investigators had developed sophisticated techniques that allowed them to work with antibodies. They could test for them, understand and measure their effects, and even use them as investigative tools. Goethe observed that one searches where there is light. We knew a great deal about antibodies; there was light there. I myself was trying to find antibodies to tumor antigens.

When antibodies are *not* involved in the immune response, when immune system cells handle both the identification of targets and the killing, the response is called "cellular immunity." T lymphocytes, a type of white blood cell called T cells because they mature in the thymus, are the most important cells in cellular immunity.

It was well established that transplanted tissue, whether a skin graft or a kidney transplant, is attacked by the cellular immune system and by T lymphocytes. It seemed to me that cancerous tissue had more in common with transplanted tissue than with a bacterial infection, which generates an immune response involving antibodies.

In addition, some investigators had reported that T lymphocytes killed tumors in animal experiments. Many immunologists dismissed these experiments.

I felt differently. It was not that I lacked skepticism. Actually, I take a skeptical view of most scientific articles. Theoretically one should be able to trust all scientific literature; theoretically they report objective, observed facts. But often they do not. Unless I personally know the author, know that he or she is reliable, I am very skeptical of all but the most rigorously proven experimental results.

And how a scientist interprets papers has enormous impact on his or her work. Einstein won his Nobel Prize not for the theory of relativity but for explaining the photoelectric phenomenon. The phenomenon was well known and hundreds of articles had been written about it, but none had explained it. Einstein sliced through an enormous amount of information to get the answer. When asked what he considered his major scientific talent, he said it was his ability to look at a large number of experiments and select the very few that were correct, ignore all the rest, and build a theory on the right ones. His talent, he said, was deciding which data were right and which were wrong.

Few papers—very, very, very few—are the product of fraud.

But I think as many as 30 percent of scientific articles contain results or conclusions that are wrong and are not reproducible. A good many more stretch their conclusions far beyond what their evidence will support.

The reason is that too often investigators allow themselves to be fooled. Perhaps they haven't designed the experiment properly and don't have both a positive and a negative control. Or perhaps they want a result so badly that it influences their judgment. Often a result depends on a subjective measurement, and unconscious bias can affect measurements of, say, the size of a tumor difficult to feel or the evaluation of the extent of swelling at an injection site. Wanting a particular answer can sometimes lead to getting it. Bias can also enter into the decision about which data to discard. A scientific article may involve work that covered many years and hundreds of experiments, and one cannot report all experimental results. But is the data in the article representative of all the experiments, or only the ones that seem to confirm the hypothesis? Investigators can easily rationalize. "The technician forgot to change the water in mouse cage number six for four days," they might say to themselves, "and that's why those mice died. So we shouldn't count them in the results."

Good scientists are aware of these problems and do not yield to them, but not all people who do science are scientists.

All scientists have to make judgments about which technical articles to use as foundations for their own work, which ones to discard and which ones to believe. To a considerable extent, what they achieve depends as much upon these judgments as upon their own experiments. I chose to believe the articles that reported that T lymphocytes, T cells for short, killed cancers in animals.

T cells were, I believed, what I was looking for.

CHAPTER FIVE

On the wall of my office are individual photographs of each of the sixty fellows who have trained under me, except for Norman Wolmark. He alone has never sent me one. Considering what he went through here, I can hardly blame him. Yet his sardonic wit and almost bitter sense of the absurd made him the perfect person to help in my first efforts to work with T cells. It was a high-risk project, but if it succeeded the payoff would be enormous.

What I had in mind was based on work recently done by an English scientist named M. O. Symes, and some discussions I had had with my friend Dave Sachs, who was working in transplantation. We bounced ideas off each other constantly, and played squash and had dinner together once a week. Symes had done something strange. He had injected pieces of a human bladder cancer into the mesentery of the intestinal tract of pigs in an attempt to immunize them against the tumor. He then harvested the pig lymphocytes and infused them into patients with bladder cancer. He claimed some tumors had regressed.

It was bizarre and made little sense. Virtually all of the immune reaction of the pigs should have been directed against the vast differences between species, and not against the minute and subtle differences—if any—between normal and cancerous human cells.

But at the time, in 1976, both our clinical and lab work in immunotherapy were disappointing. The randomized protocols with BCG were demonstrating its ineffectiveness, and the complications and pain BCG caused our patients made it worse than futile.

My intuition remained firm that stimulating an immune response to cancer was a valid approach, but nothing I was trying worked. In the lab I was still confronting the nightmare—that no immune response to cancer existed in humans. I hoped to resolve this by finding antibodies to tumor antigens; if antibodies existed, then the immune system was by definition responding—however feebly and ineffectively. It would prove that my approach to the disease, in principle at least, could work. A few months before Norm Wolmark arrived, George Parker, a fellow in my lab, and I believed we had detected antibodies to a mouse tumor, but these observations were tenuous.

I felt like a dog trying to bite a basketball. If only I could somehow get leverage, I felt progress was possible. But how could I achieve that?

In fact, the only progress we were making anywhere was in our clinical trials with sarcoma, cancers of the soft tissues. These trials were emotionally draining, and even our progress only reinforced the need for something better. We were trying to determine whether the traditional treatment of amputation of a limb improved long-term survival rates of sarcoma victims, as compared to the limb-sparing local excision of a tumor combined with radiation therapy. This was similar to work being done by others in breast cancer, comparing radical mastectomies and lumpectomies. Eight years after our study began, it ended; the survival rates were identical. Amputation has now been replaced by limb-sparing surgery as the standard treatment for sarcoma.

These trials marked a difficult experience for me. In getting informed consent from our patients, we had to tell them that we did not know whether an amputation or a local operation was better for them, and ask them to agree to have their treatment decided by chance. Many patients refused to enter the protocol. Those who did I came to know intimately. As a resident at the Brigham, rotating from service to service, one lived one's life in two-month blocks and did not follow patients for extended periods of time. In the sarcoma trials we followed our patients for years, through the entire course of their treatments and follow-ups. I soon learned how both gratifying and painful this intimacy can be.

I recall two of our earliest patients vividly. Emily Reinaud was a professor of art at a Midwestern university. She had undergone surgery to resect an abdominal sarcoma; the surgeon told her he had gotten all of the cancer and that her belly was free of disease. At the time we only suspected what the sarcoma trials, which lasted several years, demonstrated: Approximately half the time the surgeon failed to remove all the local cancer.

This particular case was a rare cancer and the operation had been a very difficult one, complicated by problems with bleeding. In the face of this, I doubted that her surgeon, who was a general surgeon and not a cancer expert, had had the persistence to explore as fully as he should have. I advised her to have another exploratory operation. Her doctor advised her not to. She rejected my recommendation and went home. A month later, however, she changed her mind and returned. I operated and did find another tumor, lodged on the vena cava, a main blood vessel. With great difficulty, we removed part of the vena cava.

That Christmas she sent me an exquisite glass paperweight, promised to send me one every year as long as she was alive, and hoped my collection would be a large one. I now have fifteen beautiful works from Emily. Receiving one is a special thrill.

I remember Sharon Watson just as vividly. She was a doctor at NIH, a fellow on another service. Young and athletic, she and her husband, a physicist, were avid bikers and hikers. She felt a lump in the muscle of her abdominal wall one day and came to me. It was sarcoma. I operated and removed it. But if one cancer cell escapes the knife, it can grow into fresh tumors. Several months later she came to me and said she had noticed that she could not push on her bike pedal quite as hard as usual. The cancer had recurred. When she died eight months later, her husband asked everyone to leave the room. We did, and he locked the door, combed her hair, fixed her up on a pillow, and played the guitar to her for an hour.

These trials reminded me that the knife was often not enough.

We had to find a way to attack all the cancer—every single cancer cell in the body. Surgery could not do that. The immune system could.

Symes gave a seminar at NCI about his work with pig lymphocytes. He seemed excitable and unable to provide the kinds of details about his work that would convince me his claims were real. But I was desperate and the experiment seemed at least a start in the direction of obtaining antitumor cells for human therapy.

When one does not know how to solve a problem, sometimes it is necessary to attack it by stumbling about in its general vicinity, scratching at its edges, or even running headlong into it in the hope that one's aggression will itself either force open a crack that allows one to peer inside or create new angles from which to view the problem and possibly gain a new insight. Pasteur once observed, "Chance favors the prepared mind." I prefer a comment made in passing by Franny Moore on rounds and which is hanging on the wall of the lab: "Chance cannot enter the prepared mind unless the mind is at work."

It was with this intent that I began to work with the pigs.

There was a history of interactions between animal immune systems and humans. Horses, for instance, were used for decades to produce tetanus antitoxins. Tetanus is a deadly disease, largely eradicated in the developed world, caused by bacteria that secrete a toxin; the toxin can cause lockjaw, respiratory paralysis, and death. Scientists learned to infect horses with the bacteria, wait for their immune systems to develop antibodies—called antitoxins—and extract these antibodies from the horses' blood. Persons suffering from tetanus received injections of these antibodies, which physically bound to the toxin, in effect handcuffing it and making it harmless. In recent years tetanus vaccine has largely replaced the horse antitoxin, but it was effective.

I needed T cells that would react against cancer. There was no way to get large numbers from patients, and T cells could not be grown in culture. The pigs, after being immunized as Symes had done, could provide these T cells in large numbers. And although patients' own immune systems would certainly reject T cells from pigs, this rejection would take time to develop. Meanwhile, perhaps the pig cells could do some good.

Another reason to proceed was that transplants of cells and tissue from one species to another were becoming very interesting as immunologists began exploring the possibility of using other-than-human sources of organs for human transplantation. Dave Sachs was becoming deeply involved in the field. These experiments might teach us a lot.

So I decided to proceed, and if the lab was going to do it, I intended to do it properly. Norm had hoped to do laboratory research, possibly working with antibodies and antigens. The pig experiments would involve surgery, and Norm's surgical experience surpassed that of the other fellows. He had just finished his surgical residency. Unfortunately for Norm, he did not get the opportunity to do the antiseptic, laboratory science he wanted. He worked hard anyway.

The pigs lived contentedly in a separate building, the "large-animal facility," which was about a quarter of a mile from the Clinical Center and connected to it by an underground tunnel. The tunnel was dimly lit, a good fifteen feet wide, and it seemed to run forever. It just about did, connecting much of the campus. Wandering through the tunnel system, one felt as if one had entered an H. G. Wells novel, complete with moorlocks, netherworld, and secret doors and unknown passageways leading into the earth's bowels. Steam pipes hissed overhead and forklifts and small trucks trundled by, carrying freight or dragging a small train of carts. Judging by the stares of these tunnel denizens, we must have been the only doctors who ever passed by; no doubt we made an odd sight in our procession on our way to operate, pulling behind us dollies loaded with tissue culture flasks, bottles of medium, and the specialized equipment we needed.

The animal facility was equipped with its own operating rooms, X-ray facility, pathology lab, scrub room, and O.R. nurse. It looked in fact like a first-class hospital O.R.; it simply did not smell like one. The actual work involved three surgical procedures. First, in the Clinical Center labs we resected tumors from rats and mice—and ultimately patients. We then performed formal laparotomies on the pigs—hoisting them onto an operating table, anesthetizing and intubating them, scrubbing down exactly as we would for any operation under antiseptic conditions—and placed small slices of these tumors into the intestinal mesentery of the pigs, an area where large lymph nodes exist. After waiting several weeks for an immune response to develop, we harvested the nearby lymph nodes. Norm also performed splenectomies on the pigs. (Pigs, and man, can easily survive without spleens.) We took excellent care of the pigs, both before any procedure and postoperatively.

The pigs, however, did not seem to appreciate this good care, and they quickly taught us that they are interesting and intelligent animals. Oddly enough, they reminded me of my first scientific experiments with hamsters. Hamsters are malleable for an initial experiment, but they remember. Later, whenever the investigator walks by their cage, they flip onto their backs, bare their fangs, and pull back their claws—waiting to revenge themselves. The pigs also cooperated initially in our investigations, but as Norm once said, "If you operate on a dog, it'll lick your hand. If you operate on a pig, it will remember and try to kill you."

Even though we worked with small pigs, some still weighed hundreds of pounds. Norm had to corral them and put them in a sort of wooden fence in the corridor, which quickly became inundated with pig feces. As he once said, "I not only did the experiment but got a critique on it immediately."

Finally, back in the lab, Norm isolated lymphocytes from the nodes. This was not clean work. Particularly when he was working with spleens, his area resembled an abattoir. He mashed up the spleens, passed them through mesh, then mixed them in solution to isolate individual cells. Blood was everywhere. The sight would become a common one in our lab.

Meanwhile Norm proceeded, perfecting techniques and measuring results. Sometimes working with the pigs seemed a joke to others—and sometimes even to some of those in my lab. People wandered by the lab, watched Norm mashing up spleens, blood everywhere, asked what he was doing, and were uniformly astounded. "Surely you don't think this will work," many commented.

To raise morale in the lab, I hosted a huge pig barbecue in my backyard. Even that ran into problems. My father, the Orthodox Jew, would have been repulsed had he known. The day scheduled for the barbecue, it rained; the pig had to stay in my cellar in a vat of brine overnight. When we finally placed it on the spit, we did not roast it long enough. Except for the outer portions, it was raw.

And yet our work was serious. The only immunotherapy tried at NIH prior to this had been scratching BCG bacteria into the skin. Now we were keeping a herd of pigs, performing major operations on them, drowning a lab with their blood. We were intent.

And now we were about to give their lymphocytes to our first patient.

Linda Karpaulis was pregnant with her third child when her thigh began to bother her. Her physician diagnosed an undifferentiated sarcoma, a particularly vicious cancer. Patients come to NIH only through referrals from other physicians. When we begin a protocol, physicians in private practice are informed of our interest in having patients in particular clinical situations referred to us. It can sometimes be difficult to get doctors to refer their patients to us if the disease already has a standard treatment with a reasonable prognosis. We have had to abandon more than one research protocol because we could not get a patient population sufficient to make the study worthwhile. But when doctors feel they have nothing to offer their patients, or when standard treatment is particularly difficult, they willingly send patients to us.

Now we were actively seeking patients for our randomized sarcoma protocol. Standard treatment often required mutilating operations, and even then the prognosis was poor. No doctor likes to perform these operations, especially on young people. We had many referrals.

Ms. Karpaulis was young, only twenty-four then, and her physician referred her to us. Short and compact, she was from Pennsylvania, Caucasian, and poor. With her hair pulled back she had a harried, tough, school-of-hard-knocks look. Nothing made her smile. And yet there was an enormously appealing quality about her.

She had a stoicism that went beyond courage; it was a kind of innocence. Everyone who met her wanted to protect her. She was struggling against both life and her disease without knowing the power of her adversaries. Through all her difficulty she never showed emotion. She reacted hardly at all, to anything, except when her children entered the conversation. Then she became fierce; one could imagine her killing to defend her children—they were all she cared about. But we had no good news.

I brought her into my office and explained the options. She came alone; her husband stayed home. She had a very aggressive cancer. The standard treatment was to amputate her leg and give adjuvant chemotherapy. Even then she had only a 40 percent chance of surviving five years. The alternative was local excision of her tumor along with radiation treatment and chemotherapy. We hoped this would improve the quality of life of patients with sarcoma. But we did not know at that point if local excision had a comparable survival rate. That was what we were trying to find out.

If she entered the protocol, her treatment would be selected by chance. If she decided not to enter the protocol, she could choose either amputation or local excision and have it done elsewhere.

"Those aren't very good choices, are they?" she said flatly. There was nothing I could say. A moment later she agreed to enter the protocol and signed the informed consent.

She randomized to amputation. I did the hemi-pelvectomy myself. This is a painful, mutilating operation, involving an amputation at the hip that includes the hipbone itself. Postoperatively she seemed strong. But what was she thinking? She was twenty-four years old with three small children and one leg. How could she take care of them? NIH offered patients both counseling and extensive support structures.

"Possibly we can help," I said. Did she want some help?

"I'll manage."

"Are you sure? There's actually quite a lot we can do."

"I'll be all right."

She gave back nothing. She left the hospital and returned monthly for chemotherapy. Then she disappeared, missing numerous follow-up visits.

A year and a half later she came back. She had given birth to another child. She had not kept her follow-up appointments because she had feared we would have forced her to abort the fetus or given her therapy, which would have risked hurting it. We would have done neither. For a person in her situation, living on the edge as she was, any decision about a child is a personal, not a medical, one.

Still, she seemed to be coping well and felt wonderful physically. She had returned only because she wanted a prosthesis. Her desire for a prosthesis was a good sign, indicating that she wanted to get on with her life. Perhaps it had something to do with her image of herself as a mother, or simply as a whole person. Regardless of the reason, it seemed a declaration that she was determined to take charge of things. We were thrilled at her apparent good health and spirits.

As part of the routine follow-up visit I ordered a series of tests. I didn't expect to see any problem when I reviewed her chest X ray. There was a problem. The cancer had returned in her lungs. She underwent more chemotherapy but her X rays did not show improvement. Although to the casual observer she seemed healthy and energetic, her situation was worsening quickly.

I discussed a treatment plan with her. We would perform a thoracotomy on one side of her chest. Our hope was that we would not find many lesions. If we could remove them all, then two weeks later we would open the other side of her chest and try to make her disease-free by cutting out all the cancer we could find. If there were not too many cancer deposits and we could remove them all, there was a chance, a slim one, of curing her.

Patients with four or fewer lung metastases have a 20 percent chance of being cured. If they have more than six metastases, they have almost no chance.

"It's possible, however," I said, "that we will not be able to take out all the cancer. If that happens there is something else very experimental that we've never done but that we can try, if you are interested."

I explained the pig experiment to her and asked if she would consider trying that if the surgery failed. She said she wanted to try anything.

In early October Wayne Flye, our chief chest surgeon, performed the thoracotomy. About thirty minutes after starting the case, Flye paged me and asked me to come to the O.R. Fifty percent of the time the surgeon finds more cancer in the lungs than the X rays reveal. This was one of those times; her lungs were thick with small tumors. We counted twenty-five nodules between one and ten millimeters in diameter.

Most surgeons would have simply closed. It was pointless to resect them—her lung was certainly laced with dozens of other nodules not yet large enough to see, and her other lung would be similar. Flye asked what I wanted to do. She was so young. There was something unholy about closing and leaving the cancer. We cut them out. We already had a pig ready for a laparotomy; if we were to try the therapy with the lymphocytes, the slices of her tumor would have to be fresh. I called Norm in the animal facility to tell him to begin the operation on the pig. A surgical resident carried the tumor specimens down the long underground tunnel to Norm, and he sewed them into the pig's mesentery.

On October 31, 1977, I submitted a protocol to the NCI Clinical Research Committee seeking expedited permission to perform a clinical experiment infusing immunized pig lymphocytes into patients with advanced cancer. November 7 we received approval.

On November 14, I went over the informed consent with Ms. Karpaulis in detail, explaining that we had never done it before. But there was nothing else to try. I added, "There may be some danger but we will be right there."

72

She said, "My oldest kid is six years old. I want to see him grow up."

A moment later she continued, "I'm not very religious." Unsaid, her message seemed to be that she was putting her faith in me.

The next day at 12:15 we gave her 5 ccs of the pig lymphocytes intravenously. It was a test dose. She showed no reaction. We proceeded. She received a total of five billion cells intravenously. An hour and forty minutes later she developed chills. Twenty minutes later her temperature shot up to 38° Celsius, then 39°, which is 103.2° Fahrenheit, but soon returned to normal. The next day hives erupted near the site of the infusion. One day later, not quite forty-eight hours after she received the cells, she was discharged.

When she returned for follow-up, CAT scans revealed new lesions on the right side and bone metastases. The treatment had done no good. We gave her more chemotherapy. The disease progressed. In May she underwent a second thoracotomy. There were too many nodules to resect. This time the surgeon closed leaving the cancer intact.

She was dying and had little money—in fact, she was on welfare. Again I tried to talk to her and again she showed no emotion. But one day in the hospital I saw her with a small tape recorder. I asked her what it was for.

"My children are too young to remember me," she said. "I'm recording messages for them to listen to when they're older. I want them to know their mother."

It was a desperate cry for existence, to say, *I counted. I made a mark. I was here.* Perhaps participating in our experiment made her feel that she had made a mark, too. I hoped so.

She was concerned about dying—about pain, about suffering. At least I could reassure her about that. It was a conversation with which I was already too familiar, and with which I would become even more familiar.

"We haven't given up," I told her, "but it may not be possible for us to control the disease." I hesitated for a moment, then continued. "Do you have any questions? About anything? About anything at all . . ."

She was lying in bed and turned her head to the side, away from me, then asked softly, "What's it like?"

We wouldn't allow her to struggle for breath, I told her. There would be no sense of suffocation. There wouldn't be any pain either. We had drugs that could reach any pain, no matter how deep. If it came to that, the drugs would make her sleep more and more. Finally she would just sleep.

Linda Karpaulis did not die in our hospital. She went home and slowly deteriorated.

Later, Norm expressed the reaction of all of us: "She was an extremely courageous individual. I've since come to understand that's not a unique phenomenon among patients with no hope of a cure for metastatic disease. If we didn't provide her with hope, we gave her a sense that she was contributing, which to her was important."

She tolerated the treatment very well. So did the five others who received it. It had no effect on their cancers.

Norm Wolmark devoted two years of serious effort to this pig work, but almost everything about it was a failure. It taught us only that people can tolerate the infusion of large numbers of lymphocytes, up to thirteen billion cells. Norm wrote four papers about his experiments which were summarily rejected by journals. The lab is a lonely place. Sometimes looking foolish has nothing to do with the logic or power of an idea itself, but only with intellectual fashions of the moment. Some people refuse to look foolish even to themselves; they will not pursue anything that contradicts conventional wisdom. But if one is to make progress, one must be prepared to look foolish. At my request, Norm had the courage to do what seemed foolish.

I have always felt badly that Norm could never publish any of this work and I remain convinced that in some ways it was ahead of its time. Today, with the supply of human organs for transplants far short of demand, experimenting with other species has become an important area of transplantation immunology. Organ transplants between species, for example, between primates and pigs, are now being performed. In the not too distant future I expect experiments to be conducted on man, and as I write this Dave Sachs has just left NIH to set up a center at Harvard to study transplants between species.

The experience did no harm to Norm, now chief of surgery at Montefiore Hospital in Pittsburgh. And his sense of the absurd is stronger than ever. His office, which is three or four times the size of mine, lies at the end of a long corridor and visitors must be screened by two secretaries to get there, which shields him well from casual interlopers. Even so, he keeps his office door locked, sits at his desk far from the door, and buzzes people in.

By the time Norm was ready to leave, our lab was exploring a new idea, one that might allow us to use our patients' own lymphocytes against their cancers. My memory of his last few months was of him wearing a wistful look, watching other investigators grow mouse and human cells in antiseptic, pristine white-tabled conditions, doing the kind of hard science he had hoped to do, then turning back to his abattoir. In regular lab meetings each investigator submitted his latest findings for criticism; at least one former colleague recalls Norm as being the most acerbic of the critics. Norm says now, "I thought everything has its time. I wouldn't say I was disappointed but I recognized the significance of having arrived at the lab two years too soon. What they were doing when I left—it was very exciting. I could see its potential immediately."

PART TWO

FIVE IFS AND THEN

CHAPTER SIX

In September 1976, just as I began the pig effort, Robert Gallo and two scientists working in his lab, Doris Morgan and Francis Ruscetti, published a paper in *Science*, one of the most prestigious journals in the world. Their interest was leukemia—cancer of blood cells—and they had been trying to grow long-term cultures of human leukemia cells for use in future experiments. But to their dismay, they found that instead they were growing healthy human T lymphocytes. They explored this phenomenon enough to identify a protein that they believed caused the growth and called it "T Cell Growth Factor," which later became known as Interleukin-2 or IL-2. Although they published the finding, they did not pursue the immunologic aspects of their discovery aggressively, instead returning to their original area of leukemic cells. (Ultimately this led to Gallo's discovery of the first human leukemia virus, which caused a rare T-cell leukemia.)

Gallo's paper was exciting. Until its publication, immunologists did not believe it possible to grow T cells in vitro—in a laboratory culture—for more than a few days, and even then only when they were stimulated with antigens. Morgan, Ruscetti, and Gallo had grown them for as long as nine months without antigens. For me this had enormous potential significance.

T lymphocytes are the more common of the two chief kinds of lymphocytes, beginning development in the bone marrow before maturing in the thymus and accounting for approximately 70 percent of all lymphocytes. B lymphocytes, which begin development in the bone marrow and mature there, account for about 25 percent of all lymphocytes; when stimulated, they transform themselves into antibody-producing factories.

T cells divide into two major sub-types: killer cells and helper cells. Helper cells regulate activity in cellular immunity, which primarily involves T cells, and control the ability of B cells to make antibodies. (The AIDS virus destroys helper T cells, preventing the body from defending itself against infections.) Killer T cells of course kill, and they do so by binding highly specific receptors on their surface to antigens.

T cells are shaped like a somewhat off-center tennis racket; they are smooth and shimmering under a microscope when alive. When they are dead and fixed under a scanning electron microscope, they resemble floating mines—globular cells with thousands of tiny spikes protruding from the surface. If the proper antigen binds with the proper receptor, a process begins that can end in the explosive death of a foreign cell. But although a T cell may have thousands of receptors protruding from its surface, each of these receptors is identical. Thus, each T cell will bind with only one kind of antigen.

T cells emerge from the thymus fully mature, fully differentiated, themselves an end product and in their own way as mature and differentiated as a finger. This explains why immunologists did not consider it possible to grow them. No one can take cells from a finger and generate a new finger. Similarly, it was thought that T cells probably could not be grown in vitro.

These findings seemed significant to me, yet I did not pick up on them immediately. It wasn't that there was any reason to doubt the science—I knew Gallo; he headed another branch at NCI and did first-rate work. But I was distracted, if not consumed, primarily by my efforts to find antibodies for tumor antigens. Other work was also continuing in my department—the BCG and sarcoma clinical trials—and the pig lymphocyte work was beginning.

The article also left many unanswered questions. For example, nothing in it suggested these cells could maintain their function and kill after being grown in culture.

Still, if I did not attend properly to Gallo's work, ideas did begin to ferment in my mind. If I actually could grow T cells in the laboratory and they could maintain their killing function, then for the first time I might dissect—and manipulate—elements of the cellular immune system reactive against cancer in ways that previously had been impossible.

Ten months after Gallo's paper appeared, Kendall Smith, who was at Dartmouth and on his way to becoming the world's expert on IL-2, and his post-doctoral fellow Steve Gillis published an article in *Nature,* another influential scientific journal, about using IL-2 to grow mouse T cells. This not only confirmed Gallo's work with human T cells but opened the door to experimentation; for obvious reasons one could experiment with mice in ways impossible with people. Back then I had not heard of Smith, but his paper clearly represented good science. It registered strongly on me.

A few weeks after its publication there was a small meeting at Oxford to discuss manipulating the immune response to cancer. I rarely attend large conferences; if I go at all it is to give a talk and leave. This was different. Only forty-five people were in attendance and they were among the best immunologists in the world.

Oxford is a timeless place. I had never been there before. There were no students at the university during the conference, only we scientists, and we lived in the dormitories and shared rooms. No special efforts were made to make us comfortable. Yet we were wonderfully comfortable. The greens, the quiet streams that divided the campus, the medieval architecture, the dons walking about in strange gowns created a feeling almost of divinity, of ancient monks arguing about ancient gods. Though we were discussing the most modern aspects of science, we all felt a connection to a thirst for understanding that began with the dawn of man. And "discussing" is the right word. While there were formal presentations—almost exclusively about antibodies and little about T cells—the schedule allowed extensive free time for intense, casual conversation and the trading of ideas. London's Av Mitchison, an expert on cellular immunity, organized the conference. Richard Gershon, a brilliant immunologist who chain-smoked and died of lung cancer a few years later in his late thirties, came from Yale. I talked at length with George Klein and Peter Alexander, both already famous for their work. A dozen others exchanged ideas with me, especially Hermann Wagner, a German who was extending many of Smith's experiments.

The conversations, the fermentation of my own ideas, the recent papers combined to make me wonder: *Let's say Gallo and Smith are right. Let's say you can grow differentiated T lymphocytes using their method. T cells are killers. Then what?*

And I began to get excited.

From Oxford I flew directly to another scientific conference in Japan along with two NCI immunologists, Bill Terry, who headed the immunology branch, and Rich Hodes. Rich began to brief me on the latest, very new findings about T cells, most of it work done by Lloyd Old and Ted Boyse in New York. It was after midnight. The lights were dimmed so people could sleep but we kept talking. Severe turbulence over the North Pole interrupted us. Flying does not frighten me but I remember feeling a strange sense of urgency. I kept demanding of Rich that he tell me more, tell me more, gesturing with my hands. Suddenly I realized my urgency came from wanting to learn everything before the plane crashed.

In Japan I could not sit through any of the talks. I felt a visceral need to begin a new series of experiments. I had to get back to the lab. Eighteen hours after my plane touched down in Osaka, I flew back to Washington.

I returned from Oxford and Japan on September 17, 1977. Immediately I began preparing a new experiment, unlike any I had performed before. I tried to make IL-2 myself from mice. The papers by Gallo and Smith gave general guidance as to how to make it, but neither scientist knew how to produce it very well. So I followed their general instructions and my own intuition and produced our lab's first IL-2. On September 26, I added it to two different cultures of T cells.

Then I waited.

One culture started with 10,000 cells. After five days it had

300,000 cells. The other started with 100,000 cells and after five days grew to 1.2 million cells. The T cells had grown!

They soon stopped growing and the cultures crashed, but the experiment suggested that the approach might work. I quickly began setting up more experiments.

It was at this time that my wife and I had planned to go away. For months I had promised this to Alice. We have an unusual relationship.

Once, I was home with my youngest daughter, Naomi, when the hospital called. One of my patients was in a dire situation. I had to come immediately. Alice was due back at any moment but my daughter was too young to leave alone. I would have to take her to the hospital with me. Just then Alice called. She had been in an accident. A tractor trailer had made an illegal turn and destroyed our car. She was fine, she assured me, but shaken.

"Where are you?" I asked. She was close by. "I'll be right there."

I arrived at the scene. The top of the car had gone underneath the trailer and was crushed. It seemed miraculous that Alice had not been killed. I asked her again if she was hurt, and she again assured me that she was not physically injured, only terrified.

"Good," I said. "Listen, can you take care of Naomi? I've got to get to the hospital. My patient's in much worse shape than you are."

I left the two of them standing there, Naomi excited by the destruction and the bustle and the approaching sirens, and Alice glaring with an odd mixture of bewilderment and amusement.

Few people, men or women, would tolerate a spouse doing that but Alice is independent, strong, and able to handle a crisis coolly. She always could, which was one reason she became head nurse of the Brigham emergency room at such a young age. In the life-threatening situations that so often occur in emergency rooms, she would routinely set up equipment for procedures long before the doctor realized he would perform them. Young doctors used to seek her advice and guidance back then. Bruce Weintraub, a friend now at NIH, recalls having just graduated from Harvard Medical School, which teaches theory well but does not emphasize practice, and beginning his internship at the Brigham when a patient came into the emergency room suffering from intestinal bleeding. Bruce needed to insert an Ewal tube into the stomach. Suddenly the tube was in his hands. But he did not know whether to insert it through the mouth or the nose—most tubes are inserted through the nose but an Ewal is larger than most tubes. He held the tube in the general proximity of the nose and looked at Alice, who was standing at the foot of the bed. She gave a gentle and subtle shake of her head no. He held it near the mouth, and Alice nodded yes. He has remained forever grateful.

Alice has taken charge of many parts of our life—doing our taxes, arranging for home repairs, even putting gas in my car—to leave me free for my work. For this her friends have criticized her, telling her she has become subservient to me. That is not an accurate depiction of our relationship and omits such facts as her job as managing editor of the *Journal of Immunotherapy*. If the depth and intensity of her commitment to me seems unusual, I am equally committed to her. If we spend little time together, that time is precious and sacred. Our dinners together are inviolate, as are the Sunday evenings when we go to movies together. And then there are the few times we get away.

For months we had planned to take a long weekend at the end of September and head for the eastern shore of Maryland, alone. We, or rather Alice, had already arranged the logistics of baby-sitters, and we had looked forward to having empty beaches and the ocean to ourselves. It wasn't often that we went on a holiday, not even once a year, but when we did we wanted solitude.

But I had just begun the first experiments with IL-2 in what could become an entirely new direction for me. The data emerging from the experiments, inconclusive as it might have seemed to another scientist, was almost overwhelming to me. I could not get the experiments out of my mind. The possibilities they presented were too enormous. To leave the laboratory then, to take a long weekend, was impossible.

The long weekend collapsed into one night away. Early Saturday morning I arrived at the hospital. In midafternoon Alice picked me up and we left for the ocean.

Still, thoughts of the experiment and the ideas generated at Oxford were swirling through my mind. I began to talk about them as soon as we left. Alice listened intently.

My thoughts were inchoate at first, but as I talked on they seemed to form a pattern revolving around IL-2. I talked of all the experiments I might try to do with it and where they might all lead. Gradually the pattern seemed to form a plan. Alice has an intuitive ability to penetrate to the heart of an issue and asked an occasional brief question. Under her prodding the pattern came into sharper and sharper focus. I talked for two and a half hours straight and finally had nothing more to say. But Alice did.

"It seems to me," she said, her eyes staring straight ahead down the road, "that you've got five 'ifs' and a 'then.'"

I laughed at first, then thought more deeply about what she had said. She was right. She had taken the diffuse thoughts about an experimental path and organized them in a precise way. There were dozens of small questions but five large ones.

If we could grow T cells from both animals and humans in culture and they maintained their killing activity, and

If those same T cells grown in culture could be infused into an animal, and they maintained their killing activity inside the animal, and

If we could next find cells in tumor-bearing animals—animals and people with cancer—that attacked their cancers, grow those cells, and they also maintained their killing activity in culture, and

If those cells could be infused back into animals, where they still killed cancers, and

If we could do the same thing in humans . . .

"That's a lot of ifs," Alice said coolly.

But her coolness marked less any skepticism than an effort to restrain her own enthusiasm. Both she and I knew the next step, although neither of us allowed ourselves to express it. It is not something I would say even in private. It is not something I would

85

allow myself even to think. But it was the goal. Assuming that one after another each of the *ifs* was satisfactorily answered in the affirmative, logic forced us inevitably to one conclusion:

Then we could cure cancer.

CHAPTER SEVEN

My plan was simple. I wanted to find T cells in a patient's body that killed cancers, remove them from the body, grow them in culture into immense numbers, and infuse them back into the patient. The T cells would then devour the cancer.

My few experimental attempts to grow T cells with IL-2 and the long conversation with Alice had ignited in me a new intensity. All mention of the work that had consumed me—using antibodies to prove tumor antigens existed—disappeared abruptly from my lab notebooks, replaced entirely by this new series of experiments. I was determined to make these experiments work.

And experiments rarely just work; an investigator must make them work. In this sense—making something work—surgery and science are alike. The surgeon performing an operation needs to be careful but cannot be timid. A surgeon must make his or her moves, especially difficult ones, with confidence. Unless the surgeon believes the operation is the right one to perform, he or she will too readily compromise and back down when difficulties arise. Similarly, if a scientist does not believe an experimental series will work, then the chances are great that it will not. Without confidence one will abandon the experiments after a few failures, instead of immersing oneself in them, wrapping oneself at all hours in thoughts about them, reviewing every variable and every reagent for ideas about adjustments to make that might solve the problems that inevitably arise. One must be willing to commit everything to one's plan. I was prepared to direct all the resources at my command to exploring the five *ifs*, the five separate elements of my hypothesis.

My office has two doors. The door to the left opens onto another office with secretaries and administrative files. Outside this area and twenty paces farther to the left is another corridor; this corridor is a hospital ward and on it are my patients.

But the door to the right of my office opens directly onto the laboratory, and I consider my office part of the lab. Since every inch of office space takes an inch away from work space in the lab, the office is as small as I can tolerate. There is no room for a coffee table; there is not even an armchair or a sofa. A television monitor by my desk allows me to observe the operating room. Next to it is a computer. A small conference table is jammed between my desk and a blackboard, which is constantly filled with step-by-step plans for the most current experiments. Next to it is a screen for viewing X rays. Books cram one wall, books on molecular biology, surgery, immunology, cancer. File cases are packed with scientific articles and drafts.

My office is cluttered, and the physical sense one gets from the lab is of clutter. Space there is also tight (no matter how large the lab gets, we always outgrow it) and so the corridors are jammed with two dozen freezers and a dozen file cabinets. Sinks, computers, rows of shelves packed with bottles or books, microscopes, and workbenches fill aisles. Scattered about are torpedolike tanks of liquid nitrogen. Cardboard boxes lie about for trash; because they hold some biological waste, they will be burned. Most work is done under laminar-flow hoods, which overhang work areas and keep them sterile while leaving approximately a foot of clearance through which an investigator can reach his or her hands. The hood areas look something like an elongated bank-teller window over a kitchen countertop. Air flow under the hood is controlled to prevent even one bacterium from falling onto the work area and contaminating an experiment. Tight, compact steel desks for each investigator are squeezed into corners. Yet space is personalized; pictures of families, sometimes of patients, and cartoons are stuck into odd corners.

The lab without people present is eerie. There is constant background noise. Motors whir, keeping freezers at -180° centigrade, and computers hum. The sounds seem hollow and echoing, like something left behind but active, the purposeless work of machines.

Still, what really strikes me about the lab when I walk into it is not the equipment but the solitude. Someone is working alone at a hood performing an experiment. Someone else is slouched over a computer trying to make sense of data. People are not isolated; often two or three investigators are arguing intently over how to interpret one result, and this too is crucial to the laboratory. But ultimately when one does research one is alone, alone with one's work and one's thoughts. In my lab our thoughts had a new purpose.

At the time I began the immunotherapy effort, my own lab was small. Two fellows, both surgeons, worked directly under me, along with Sue Schwarz, the technician whom I convinced to leave Boston and come to NIH. I took Sue off everything else and put her on this one project and also hired another technician, Paul Spiess, solely for it. At the beginning the three of us did everything.

I had initially hired Sue to work in the lab Franny Moore had granted me while I was still a resident. I had asked her to come to the Brigham for a 7:00 P.M. interview, but when she arrived I was in the O.R. and could not get out until 10:30. She waited, which showed me that she wanted the job. The interview in the doctor's lounge, with me in my greens, showed me that she was intelligent and was willing to work under unusual circumstances.

Because of my hours as a surgical resident, we probably spent no more than fifteen minutes a week together. Given her independence and reliability, this suited her well.

Sue has worked with me for almost twenty years now, and over the years our cooperation and mutual respect have forged a deep bond. Yet we almost never have personal conversations; at most we skirt personal things and I know very little about her. She comes to every lab function, every picnic, every party, and often helps organize them, yet keeps her personal life entirely separate from the lab, and socializes with people outside it.

She went to Case Western Reserve University in Cleveland, applied to medical school but did not get in, and took a job in the lab of one of her professors. She liked doing research, liked the feel of the lab. The lab requires considerable manual dexterity, performing delicate operations with minute quantities of materials. Sue has golden hands. She makes quilts and has won awards for them. With her, things work. She is one of the most precise individuals I have ever worked with, yet also the fastest. Sue is a craftsman in the finest meaning of the word. One gets the sense that the workmanship itself, rather than the results of an experiment, gives her satisfaction.

Her life seems to have a fixed, well-defined quality; it is as if Sue has carefully compartmentalized everything, as if she wants things ordered enough that she can reach for things and find them in the dark. Her desk and work area are neat, tidy. One cannot push her. Sue paces herself and knows her pace well; if I ask her to perform certain assays by a certain time, she will refuse if she does not think she can do so properly. Few others in the lab will tell me no. I have learned that when she objects she is usually right, and I listen.

Because of her organizational ability, I have given her considerable authority. For years she kept the lab stocked with inventory and bargained with commercial suppliers. Many of the surgeons who come to the lab have no experience at all doing real science and she grooms them, a responsibility she takes seriously. Basically she runs the lab, and she runs it like an aristocrat.

Many people in the lab are a little afraid of Sue. She has authority because everyone knows I count on her, and she uses it, ordering scientists, for example, to clean up after themselves. If she left, I would miss her and the infrastructure of the lab would be threatened. She is a vital part of it.

If some people are a little afraid of Sue, they are amazed by Paul Spiess.

My major gauge of the inventiveness of scientists who come into the lab is how they get along with Paul. The rigid ones are bothered by him; the ones with open, creative minds enjoy being around him.

Paul has never married and is quiet, almost shy around people he doesn't know well. He lifts weights, belongs to the National Rifle Association, and is—at least by the standards of most NIH scientists—politically conservative, which means he is a moderate Republican. He is also brilliant. Unlike Sue's work area, his has a certain sloppiness about it, as if he has never quite caught up with his own ideas. On his desk one is as likely to find a book on computer logic and artificial intelligence as a copy of *The National Enquirer*. Many technicians simply perform routine tasks, like counting cells or preparing medium, which require strict adherence to procedures but little thought. Paul thinks.

After attending an exclusive private school in suburban Washington, Paul went to Johns Hopkins and majored in physics. He was always interested in science, always wanted to understand how things worked, and understand the underlying truths that make the world we know. But he left before completing college, joined the Navy, and served in Naval Intelligence in Iceland, which he describes as "the way the world was half a billion years ago—with volcanoes, ice, and green fuzzy things growing on rocks."

After the Navy he became interested in degenerative diseases and the aging process, finished college and his master's in biology at American University, started a Ph.D. program at the University of Tennessee, but stayed only one semester. Money was a problem for him. "I don't know why it costs so much to go to school," he says. "All you need to learn is a brain and a book."

Back in Washington he worked the night shift as an assembly-line supervisor in a factory making printed circuits. He was in his thirties and felt he was wasting his mind.

Paul's training is not deep, but he thinks more, has made more of a contribution to our work and had more good ideas than many of the scientists in the lab. He thinks in creative ways and has a way of talking about science in layman's terms, which puts off the more rigid scientists. Once he told me, "I don't think we know as much as we think we know. We're very empirical, like metallurgists three thousand years ago. They didn't know what an atom was, but by experimentation they made pretty good alloys. They didn't do it by understanding fundamental principles of metallurgy but by being good observers."

He often comes to me with ideas that I consider highly improbable but allow him to pursue so as not to discourage him from thinking, because others of his ideas are excellent and sometimes brilliant. His biological intuition is excellent. When Paul suggests something to me I always listen, and I listen very closely.

To Paul, his job is a search, as it is with any scientist. When I offered him a promotion to the highest professional level he can reach without a Ph.D., I pointed out that if he accepted he would no longer qualify for overtime pay. He put in so many hours, late in the evenings and on Saturdays and Sundays, the raise would end up costing him money. But the money didn't mean that much to him. It was doing science. He accepted the promotion and kept the same hours. "I'd like to do something that matters," he says. "I don't just want to use up the earth's resources and not do anything with it."

The five *ifs* provided a conceptual framework for my approach to developing an immunotherapy and broke the whole of the hypothesis into manageable parts, but offered no reason to believe it would work. There were many reasons why it might not.

Although T cells did seem able to grow in IL-2, there was no way to know whether they could grow long enough to generate the immense numbers needed. Nor could anyone know whether they would maintain their killing activity after many generations in culture. Many living things either change characteristics or lose their vitality when cultured for long periods; even wild animals can become domesticated pets. That was the first *if*.

Assuming T cells did both grow and kill in culture, no one knew whether culturing them might impart or destroy some additional quality that would prevent them from working in a living animal. That was the second *if*.

But at least those two questions could be answered definitively, yes or no.

The third *if*—finding and growing the specific T cells that reacted against the cancer, assuming such T cells existed—could take an entire scientific lifetime and still not yield an answer.

And if I did fail, how could I know whether the failure resulted from the fact that the right T cells did not exist, or from the fact that my approaches were not clever enough? Even if my hypothesis was correct, I might spend years looking for these cells and never find them.

I was well aware of the difficulties involved. Yet of all the possible approaches to immunotherapy, this one seemed to make the most sense. This one involved trying to find and grow immune cells that could kill cancer cells. Unlike the experiments with pigs or BCG, this hypothesis had a clean and elegant feel to it. It could still turn into one more demonstration of what Thomas Huxley called "the great tragedy of science: the slaying of an original beautiful hypothesis by an ugly fact." But for the first time in my life, I sensed that I could move directly and logically toward my goal.

I decided to push ahead.

And I decided something else. Normally, scientists work in a sequential fashion: they establish one premise, then build upon it for the next step; after many such steps in animals, they attempt to apply their findings to man. That was the normal way to do this. If a premise fails, if one step collapses under the weight placed upon it, one destroys only the last step. Following this path meant doing solid, even exciting science, but it could add a decade to the time needed to move experimental results from the laboratory to clinical trials.

I decided that instead of working first with animals and then man, we would work simultaneously with both. In addition, we would proceed in a staggered fashion; as soon as any progress toward solving one of the *if*s was made, we would assume ultimate success on that step and begin work on the next problem. This could cut by many years the time it would take to get to the clinic.

We began with the first question: trying to find out whether T cells would grow in culture for prolonged periods and maintain their killing activity.

I was now venturing into virgin territory. A scientist is not unlike a frontiersman trying to homestead in the wilderness. The pioneer carries nothing with him except a few basic tools, and he must be able to make more tools; if he succeeds, railroads and cities will follow. Similarly, a scientist can use tools and techniques developed by others, but the more isolated and unfamiliar the terrain, the more he or she must create: When exploring a new phenomenon, a scientist must not only make progress but often invent tools required for it and even assays that measure it. If he or she succeeds, a flood of colleagues will transform the wilderness into cities, complete with off-the-shelf supplies that reduce to minutes a task that took the pioneer months or years.

IL-2 would be the most important tool. To grow lymphocytes I was going to need large quantities of IL-2. I decided to generate it myself initially.

The first step required finding the best method to make IL-2. The basic production process involved extracting lymphocytes from the spleens of mice and mixing them in medium with a lectin, a protein derived from plants that stimulates T cells to produce IL-2 and to proliferate for three to four days. After incubation the T cells were spun out of the solution, leaving the supernatant, or "supe." The supe, which was the equivalent of soup broth after all solids have been strained out, contained the lectin, other impurities, and any IL-2 that had been secreted.

Dozens of variables affected IL-2 production, including the strain of mice from which we got the lymphocytes; incubation time before spinning out the cells; which lectin to use and how much of it; what serum and nutrients to put into the medium; even whether to grow the cells in large flasks or in small tubes.

Finding the answers involved the tedious work of preparing the supernatant many different ways and counting under a microscope T cells that had grown in it. Counting cells was our only way to measure IL-2 production; the more the cells grew, the more IL-2 the supe contained.

Paul Spiess joined the lab on October 11, 1977. Like artillery officers, we bracketed our target with experiments, read the results, and incrementally moved the brackets tighter and tighter. Paul, for example, prepared supes by using two different lectins in five different concentrations. Then we reviewed the data, picked the best lectin and lectin concentration, and repeated the experiment—no conclusion is safe when based on work that has not been reproduced. That was only one variable; there were dozens of variables and hundreds of potential combinations of them. One variable at a time, we learned how best to make IL-2. The work was laborious and time-consuming.

For a month we went absolutely nowhere. In the lab notebooks we graphed T-cell growth over time. A single piece of graph paper was large enough to cover thirteen days. Usually the cells would grow for ten days but no longer. We were desperate to get onto a second page of graph paper. Finally, in mid-November, we seemed to make some slight progress.

While trying to make IL-2, I was simultaneously working with Sue Schwarz on getting killer T cells. We mixed T cells from one strain of black mice with target cells from a strain of grey mice to generate specific killer cells.

Both of these strains were specifically bred for use in scientific experiments and they had one extremely important quality. All mice in a strain have identical genes, except for sex differences. In all experiments we use only female mice (males attack each other and the inadvertent death of one experimental mouse can distort results and destroy weeks of effort), and each black laboratory mouse was the identical twin of every other black laboratory mouse. Each grey mouse was the identical twin of all the other grey mice. The strains are the product of hundreds of generations of inbreeding; the grey mouse strain has been continuously inbred since 1909.

This inbreeding allowed us to exchange cells and tissue between animals belonging to the same strain. The immune system of one black mouse would not attack cells from another black mouse. But some T cells from black mice could recognize as foreign and attack any cell from a grey mouse.

Other scientists had developed a system to excite the particular T cells that recognized the grey mouse cells as foreign and induce this killing activity. The killing could be measured easily in a test tube. Although the basic elements of the system were well known, every lab and cell line has its own quirks. While Paul was working out the details for producing the supe containing IL-2, Sue was working out the details for producing these killer cells.

We found that after four days of exposing black mouse T cells to target cells from grey mice, we got maximum killing. The T cells were fully sensitized against cells from the grey mouse strain.

Meanwhile Paul was making progress producing the IL-2 supe.

On November 17, Sue gave Paul some killer T cells from black mice to try to grow. After they grew, we planned to test their killing ability.

If the experiment worked, then the T cells would kill the target cells they had been sensitized to but leave control cells unharmed.

We all waited.

The T cells did not grow. The IL-2 supe was not good enough. We could not test the killing.

I outlined new adjustments for Paul to try to produce better supe. The supe seemed to improve. We made more adjustments. The supe seemed more potent still.

On December 29, I had Sue again give Paul sensitized black mouse T cells. He tried to grow them again. We waited again.

The lab notebook records the result: "insufficient cells."

I was not discouraged—I was determined. We had to improve the supe more. It had to contain a higher concentration of IL-2. We made still more adjustments in the production of the supe. On January 10, Paul began growing a new batch of T cells just to test the potency of the supe.

For the first time the cells required a second piece of graph paper! They grew for nineteen days. I felt we knew how to improve the supe now and I wanted to push this progress forward even more. We made even more production adjustments.

On January 31, I decided to try once again growing Sue's black killer cells in the latest supe. It was our first really successful experiment.

The cells grew. *And they kept growing.* We had pages and pages of graph paper and finally stopped counting at 101 days. We were ecstatic.

But there was more.

On February 9, 1978, the ninth day of the culture, Sue tested the killing ability of these T cells for the first time.

In an assay that would soon become routine, she incubated target cells with chromium 51, a radioactive molecule. She then placed the killer T cells in a culture with the target cells. Live cells hold chromium 51. Dead cells release it. If the T cells killed, the dead cells would release easily detectable radioactive molecules. With a radiation counter, she measured the result.

The T cells had killed, and they had killed well.

Control cells were unharmed.

On February 14, she tried again. They killed again. On February 21, she tried again. They killed again, and again on March 2, and again on March 8. They killed and kept killing and killing. Each time control cells were untouched. Only specific target cells were killed.

We repeated the experiment with a different batch of killer cells. They also grew and repeatedly killed the target cells, and only their targets.

We repeated the experiment many times. Every Saturday I spent hours checking every cell culture, spreading them out all over the countertops, going back and forth from the incubator to the microscope. I had a huge sheet and on it tracked each culture chronologically and left detailed notes for Sue on which cultures to split—which ones were growing so well they needed to be divided—which to test, and which to leave alone. No phones rang and few people were about, but Paul always came in and worked on his project. It was quiet. There was an incredible feeling of peace doing this work, peace and wonder. I always feel a sense of awe looking into a microscope, watching live cells grow in cultures, knowing that the cells individually meant little but that together they comprised a mouse or a human being and that each individual cell was every bit as alive as a mouse or a human.

And each experiment yielded the same result. T cells could grow in IL-2 and maintain their killing function.

Excitement flooded the lab. One could feel the intensity quicken. Norm Wolmark was nearing the end of his stay and still working with the pig lymphocytes. He wanted to join our effort but it was too late. As he watched us work I had the sense of the old world looking wistfully at the new.

We had solved the first *if* in mice. Mouse killer cells would grow and still kill. Would human cells also grow and keep killing?

Not long after Sue, Paul, and I began our efforts, I pulled John Strausser, a surgical fellow, off another project and put him to work trying to do in man what we were doing in the mice.

Originally John wanted very much to do research; when I offered him a place, he had already accepted a job in Boston and sacrificed a deposit he had made on a house rental to come to NIH. But to do science one must become intimate with failure. Failure is constant and everywhere, a companion with which one shares breakfast, lunch, and dinner and which intrudes on one's enjoyment of family. A scientist must accept it and even, in a way, love it. Progress is impossible without failure; it is the foundation of success. Those who become frustrated with failure or do not learn from it cannot survive in science. John Strausser did not deal with failure well and became frustrated; toward the end, he could not wait to leave the lab and is now a plastic surgeon in Florida. He believed the IL-2 work would go nowhere and repeatedly asked to do something else.

His frustration came from his inability to keep pace with the mouse work. I had expected him to keep pace because we were first working out each problem with mice. I thought it would be relatively simple to apply to human cells whatever we achieved with murine cells. Unfortunately, the human work seemed to lag more than a pace behind.

It was not John's fault, and unanticipated problems surfaced. One was getting human blood. The NIH blood bank could not supply enough; its blood was for patients, not experiments. So John prowled our lab with a large syringe, looking for volunteers who would give blood. People in the lab sympathized with his problem but were not thrilled to see him stalking them.

A larger problem was making human IL-2. Our techniques for making murine IL-2 did not work in man, and everywhere he turned he found frustration. First, he talked with Doris Morgan, the lead author on Gallo's paper about human IL-2; she gave us some supe that contained IL-2, but she could not make it consistently either.

Next he tried to get lymphocytes from human spleens—our mouse lymphocytes came from spleens—instead of from blood drawn from the arm. So John alerted area hospitals of our need for spleens from trauma victims. A hospital would call him at 2:00 A.M. and from his home in Maryland he would dash anywhere, from downtown Washington to distant suburbs in Virginia and Maryland, to pick up the spleen while it was fresh. He grew to hate human spleens. Soon his work area was covered in blood. Flask after flask, hundreds of them, containing his various solutions of lymphocytes, lectin, and nutrients, filled every available spot in the incubators. He estimated that more than half of the flasks became contaminated. It took him months to find out that using cells from spleens made no difference. Even before that he said, "I wanted to pick up the flasks and throw them against the wall."

Next he turned to a biotechnology company. Gallo had started buying the IL-2 from Associated Biomedic Systems in Buffalo. John flew there during a winter storm and spent three days learning how the company did it. They did it better than we did and we borrowed some of their techniques, but they still did not do it very well, producing a usable batch only one out of three times.

Gradually, progressing in tiny increments, we solved the problem. The biggest single step forward came when we reasoned that human cells might differ in their ability to secrete IL-2, just as different strains of mouse cells differed in their ability to secrete it. So we decided to mix lymphocytes from several people in the same culture before stimulating them with lectin. In retrospect this seemed an obvious step to take.

Now, suddenly we were roaring ahead, and suddenly John began to get results. He quickly repeated with human cells all the work that Paul and Sue had done with murine cells. Most important, he generated killer cells from one person in the lab so they would react against target cells of another, grew them for ninety days, and repeatedly during that time tested to see if the cells maintained their ability to kill specific targets.

They did.

In both animals and man, then, in many repeated experiments, the T cells grew and maintained their specific cytotoxic activity— they were toxic to other cells. They killed. And they killed discriminately. They killed their specific targets and left other cells alone.

When John Strausser left the lab he gave me an enlarged photograph, taken through a microscope, which now hangs above the lab door. All over the photograph, everywhere one looks, human killer T cells are dividing, dividing and growing.

In the first nine days of June 1978, we submitted three scientific articles for publication, describing the best ways to produce human and mouse IL-2 and showing that T lymphocytes grown for long periods in IL-2 maintained their specific killing function. They were the first papers in what would become a long series.

Another scientist at NIH had become interested in human IL-2 when I did, and he had also tried to make IL-2. I sent him an advance copy of the paper describing our process and he came to see me. He was appalled that I had sent Strausser to Buffalo to learn techniques. It was almost as if he thought I had solved the problem unfairly.

His attitude stunned me and I almost laughed when he told me how he felt. He was a Ph.D. interested in basic immunology. For him the thrill of science was purely an intellectual one, and the thrill of the chase. He seemed to regard the problem of IL-2 as one might regard a crossword puzzle; his attitude was that it spoiled the fun to turn to the back page for the answer.

He did not know any of my patients. He had not seen Linda Karpaulis making a tape to leave her children so they would know who she was. He had not seen Sharon Watson's husband close the door to her room when she died and play the guitar for her one last time. I had.

I did not view myself as engaged in an intellectual exercise. I wanted the answer, period. Without it I could not proceed. Since my arrival at NCI, I have often had to suppress my own curiosity and choose not to pursue things that interested me because I did not believe they would take me closer to my goal.

The last of the three papers by Sue, Paul, John, and myself closed with the sentence, "Studies are in progress to . . . examine the cytotoxic potential of these cultured cells when injected *in vivo.*"

The first *if* had been answered. T cells could grow, and kill, and keep killing. They could in a test tube, anyway. Could they work in real life, in a living animal, and against cancer?

CHAPTER EIGHT

The second *if*—showing that T cells grown in culture could kill their targets when given to a living animal—was the single most unpredictable of the five elements of my hypothesis.

Because one can manipulate cells in a test tube in many ways, I had always felt confident we could use IL-2 to overcome the first hurdle. But making something work inside a living animal was entirely different. Impenetrably complex biological interactions occur in vivo, and investigators cannot manipulate conditions there as they can in a test tube. In addition, growing the cells in culture could have changed them in ways that did not affect their behavior in test tubes but could in vivo. For example, cultured T cells were four to five times larger than uncultured ones extracted from the blood. Because of their size they might get trapped in the lung and not circulate, and therefore have no impact on disease. They might even prevent the oxygenation of the blood and kill the animal.

I believed that if the hypothesis was going to collapse, it would do so in the move from test tube to animal.

The subsequent steps in my hypothesis made good scientific sense. I might be wrong, or, even if correct, I might never be able to solve the problems they presented. But the later steps were consistent with nature and the natural functioning of the immune system.

There was nothing in nature that resembled my plans to remove cells from the body, grow them in a laboratory, and put them back into the circulation of the body.

Yet if we could actually grow killer T cells that maintained their function when infused into an animal, then I believed we really would have a chance to succeed against cancer.

Maury Rosenstein joined the lab immediately after receiving his Ph.D. in immunology from Rutgers University. John Strausser's mother, a professor there, had suggested to him that he might be interested in what I was doing.

He contacted me and I invited him for an interview. To assess his creativity and the breadth of his knowledge I posed a very difficult problem for him and asked what experiments he would set up to solve it. It threw Maury off—many experienced scientists probably could not have answered the question satisfactorily—and he struggled with it. But while he struggled, as I listened to him and we talked through the problem, it seemed clear that he held within himself an abiding passion for science. It seemed to be his life. I hired him.

Maury turned out to be one of the most unselfish people I have ever known. He never seemed to care who got credit for an achievement and always seemed genuinely happy for people whose experiments were going well, even when his were not. More competitive scientists act differently; they often look jealously at those involved in exciting areas and want to jump into those areas themselves, even at the cost of abandoning their own work.

But for all Maury's sweetness he had discipline as well. He wanted to get his work done, period, regarded such maneuvering as immature, and diligently, relentlessly performed his own experiments. He accomplished what he did through hard work and by not wasting time on irrelevancies. Maury also had a unique ability to teach and to guide others, which, given the fact that most of the M.D.s in the lab had never done serious research before, was a tremendous asset.

All this made Maury a perfect model for others in the lab and helped create the atmosphere of cooperation I wanted. In the first lab meeting of each year, when new fellows arrive in July, I always make clear that everything in our lab is open to anyone on the outside. When any physician or scientist asks to visit either the lab or the clinical service, we reply with a form letter inviting them on rounds and to any lab meeting (we generally have two investigators present their latest findings each week). No one has to check with me before discussing any experiment or finding with outsiders. Our scientists can show draft papers to anyone at any stage, and they are expected to send any material we have developed to anyone who asks for it.

Unfortunately, some scientists are so competitive they operate differently. Some labs, even at NIH, close their meetings to outsiders and even to other NIH scientists. Investigators who do not want to send a reagent they have developed rarely say so flatly; instead they say it has not been fully characterized yet, or in a few more months, after more work, they will send it. But they do not.

The rise of the biotechnology industry has made this situation worse. The companies themselves often do very good science, and many university scientists have financial ties to these firms. (The government prohibits any direct financial ties for NIH scientists.) But the profit motive and the desire to protect proprietary information combine with the egos of competitive individuals to restrict the flow of information. It troubles me when a scientist knows something that could help others study cancer and refuses to share the knowledge for competitive reasons.

I think the scientific tradition of openness is contagious, just as paranoia and competitiveness are contagious. Maury was so naturally open, he influenced others in the lab, and I think in other labs, to become more open. The only conflict we ever had in his years here was when he wanted to explore things I believed were not directly enough related to the goal. There was no such conflict over his first task. He considered anything that distracted him from it an irrelevancy.

When Maury arrived, his determination and passion were such that I gave him the job of finding out whether the T cells grown in culture could kill their targets in vivo, in a live animal. Maury's task was to solve the second *if*.

Skin grafts can save the lives of burn victims, replacing tissue too damaged by heat to regenerate itself. But the grafts have to come from other parts of the victim's body. If the graft comes from another person, the victim's immune system will attack and reject it, as it will any transplant. I intended to use a well-known skin-graft model to test the ability of T cells to kill in vivo.

We would do this by grafting skin from grey target mice onto black mice. We would then treat the black mice with killer T cells that targeted the skin graft and had been grown in IL-2 supe.

If treated animals rejected the foreign skin graft faster than animals that were not treated, then we would have overcome the second hurdle. We would have shown that killer T cells grown in culture kept killing when given to an animal.

And we could then begin searching for immune system cells that recognized cancer as foreign and killed it.

Maury arrived enthusiastic and determined on July 1, 1979, immediately started work on the animal experiments, and ran into immediate frustrations.

His first had nothing to do with science. A Ph.D. among surgeons, Maury needed to learn how to perform surgery on mice. He used a model system already set up by Paul Sugarbaker. Paul was performing skin-graft experiments as part of his own studies of transplantation, not immunotherapy. He taught Maury to take skin from the ear of the donor animal and meticulously sew the graft on the recipient's back. Over the course of his experiments Maury would have to do this hundreds of times.

Initially it took him forty minutes to sew on each graft—and there were eighteen to twenty-four such procedures in each experiment—and three-quarters of them did not take. Some mice died due to the prolonged anesthesia. But after four months he could sew the grafts on in fifteen minutes and virtually every one took, at least until the immune system began attacking them.

Meanwhile Paul Spiess prepared the supernatant containing IL-2, using the spleens from hundreds of mice each week. With each preparation we thought we were making the supe more potent.

As Maury's suturing skills improved and we felt we had improved the supe, we geared up for a major experiment.

In culture, Sue sensitized killer T cells from black mice against target cells from grey mice, as she had done for our first series of experiments.

Then we grew the killer cells in the supe, and finally I injected the cells into the tail vein of the mice. This is a small vein no wider than a line of ink on a piece of paper. The injection was a delicate procedure and at the time no one else in the lab could do it consistently. I took a kind of perverse pride in the skill. The animals survived the infusion of the IL-2-grown T cells. These cells did not clog the lungs and kill the mice. That much at least was good.

Then we blinded the experiment. We did this in order to prevent unconscious bias. Reading results in many experiments—and certainly in deciding when a skin graft has been rejected—involves subjective judgment. If the person recording the result knew which animal had been treated with killer T cells, his or her judgment could be influenced by a subconscious desire to find what we were looking for. To prevent this, I had one investigator tag an ear of each mouse with a number, then write down which mice had been treated and which ones were controls. The code was kept in a sealed envelope. The mice were also randomly assigned to different cages to minimize the impact of other potential distortions, such as if the mice in one cage got an infection. A different investigator recorded the result.

Some mice rejected the skin grafts in as few as eleven days, others in as many as nineteen. The eight-day difference was a large one. If the eleven-day mice had received the killer T cells, then we would have achieved our goal: We would have shown that T cells grown in culture killed their targets when given to an animal. We would have overcome a major hurdle.

We all gathered in my office to break the code.

"The envelope, please," I said. Maury made a joke that did not hide his tension. I laughed, which did not hide mine. I opened the envelope that told us which mice had been treated and which had not.

Some of the controls had rejected the grafts in eleven days. Some of the treated mice had required many more days. The treatment had had no effect.

We were disappointed but not discouraged. Maury set up more experiments, each one with better supe and better techniques. But every experiment failed. All through the fall he failed. I could see the failure wearing on him, discouraging him. He began each experiment with enthusiasm. He ended each one with a quiet, urgent determination.

That determination showed itself one day when he was holding a mouse while I was examining its skin graft. The mouse bit him. Mice have long sharp front teeth. Their bite creates a penetrating and sudden pain. When bitten, one instinctively jerks one's hand away, which usually sends the mouse flying across the room. This can kill it, and with as few as five mice in each group, one dead mouse can distort results. And each experiment represented weeks of work.

Maury did not jerk his hand free. He let the mouse grind its teeth deeper into his finger. We had to pry the teeth loose before returning the mouse to its cage. Maury's willingness to endure pain marked how desperately he wanted the experiment to work.

But once again, when we broke the code we could see no pattern of rejection of any kind.

We changed the way we treated the mice, adjusted the way we prepared the supernatant and grew the T cells, but achieved only inklings of progress. Instead of looking forward to the code-breaking ceremony, Maury began to fear it. He began to doubt himself. Some scientists have golden hands, a touch in the lab. In their hands experiments simply work. It is hard to explain. Maury was worrying that his hands poisoned the results.

At one more failed code-breaking I watched him wince. He looked more pained than I had ever seen him. A few minutes later he went for a walk.

The NIH campus is not unlike that of a state university. Behind the Clinical Center is a stand of tall pines. Their needles carpet the ground. Maury went outside into the sunshine, soaked it in, felt the breeze blow. He stayed away for an hour, alternately sitting on a bench in the sunshine and wandering aimlessly among the grass and the evergreens.

When he returned he seemed more dogged than ever, and grim. He set up another experiment.

But why were the T cells, which killed wonderfully in test tubes, not working in the animals? What changes did we need to make to get them to work?

We had to get past this problem. The path ahead was long enough, but we could not even get started on it until we demonstrated that cultured T cells could kill their targets in vivo. As weeks turned into months, the sense of urgency and concern increased.

I believed what was blocking Maury had also blocked me earlier. Almost a year before his arrival, I had performed preliminary experiments with skin grafts with Paul Sugarbaker, who had also helped Maury set up the model. Like Maury, I had gotten negative results and puzzled over the explanation. Sugarbaker had even published a paper stating that, on the basis of these experiments, cultured T cells could not work in vivo. I had considered the experiments too preliminary to reach such a conclusion.

But we had to find an explanation—and a solution. There were dozens of possible answers. The one that seemed the most likely to me was that, although we were giving the animals many T cells, we were not giving them enough of the *right* T cells.

Less than one percent of all T cells recognized the skin graft as foreign and attacked it. We wanted to grow only this small percentage. But we were growing *all* T cells.

The problem was the lectin in the IL-2 supe.

To understand this one must understand that IL-2 makes T cells grow only if they have already been stimulated. One way to stimulate them is to expose them to their target antigen. This was how we sensitized the few T cells that recognized the skin graft.

But lectin stimulated all T cells. The supernatant containing IL-2 also contained the lectin and other impurities. When we used this supe to grow the T cells we wanted, we inadvertently grew other T cells as well. This greatly diluted and weakened the immune reaction.

I reasoned that if we used pure IL-2, if there was no lectin, then only the *right* T cells would grow because only they would be stimulated and only they would become sensitive to IL-2.

Long before Maury arrived, Sue Schwarz and I set out to test this idea by separating IL-2 from the lectin in the supe.

We went through a tedious purification process that took ten months, but by late March 1979, we could produce IL-2 with 99.99 percent of the lectin removed. This IL-2 was 300 times as potent as the raw supernatant, and a series of experiments showed that it grew the specifically sensitized T cells we wanted much better than raw supe did.

But we could not produce enough of this purified IL-2 to use it in our animal experiments. The purification process took too long and yielded only a minuscule amount of IL-2. I began looking for other ways to make large quantities of the IL-2 supe free of lectin.

Paul Spiess was struggling with this problem as well. He pointed out that we had been leaving the lectin in the spleen cultures throughout the IL-2 production process. He suggested that we add the lectin for only a short time and then rinse it away. I thought it was a terrific idea.

He suggested this on February 28, 1980. We quickly set up an in vitro experiment to try it. It showed promise. After several months refining our production method, we finally could make relatively large amounts of IL-2 supe largely free of the lectin, although not pure.

Maury immediately tried this lectin-free IL-2 in his next experiment. This seemed a major advance. With much hope we gathered in my office to break the code.

"The envelope, please," I said.

I began to read the code.

Control animals rejected the skin grafts in 15.2 days. Treated animals rejected the grafts in 12.2 days. This was statistically significant—there was a 97 percent chance that the treatment accounted for the difference and only a 3 percent chance that coincidence did. For the first experiment to yield this result was very encouraging. We were tremendously excited. But we still needed much more dramatic differences.

We made adjustments and repeated the experiment. Untreated mice still took fifteen days to reject the graft.

Animals treated with cells grown in the new IL-2 supe rejected the graft in 8.75 days.

This was excellent! The fastest a properly sewed-on skin graft can possibly be rejected, under any circumstances, is eight days.

We repeated it again. Again, untreated animals needed fifteen days to reject the graft.

Animals with treated cells rejected the grafts in 8.3 days.

The lectin-free IL-2 had worked.

For the first time I truly believed that my hypothesis not only made good scientific sense but could succeed as well. A cancer cell resembles a kind of sophisticated skin graft; it is foreign tissue, just less foreign. And for the first time I felt that, rather than floundering about in the dark hoping to hit something, we were in control of our direction and our experiments.

There was no flood of exhilaration. Too great a distance remained to be traveled to feel exhilarated. And I could still spend the rest of my scientific life searching for—and never finding—immune system cells that recognized cancer as foreign. But I did feel a new confidence that we were on the right track.

Still, before stating unequivocally that cultured T cells could kill their target when infused into animals, I needed to make certain that our model had not misled us.

The skin is a unique organ, with unique immune system sensitivities against the outside world. It was possible that skin grafts were a special case, and that T cells could attack a skin graft but still not work in the lungs or the liver or the kidney, or other internal sites where a tumor could grow.

The whole point of trying to develop immunotherapy was to find a systemic treatment that could track down and kill a single cancer cell anywhere in the body. I needed to see if T cells grown in IL-2 could function deep within the body.

To test this I began work with another animal model—one involving a cancer called FBL-3. Investigators had kept this cancer alive in laboratories for years by growing these cells in culture and transplanting them from animal to animal. During this long cultivation, the FBL-3 cancer had become almost as foreign and unnatural as a skin graft and bore little resemblance to a naturally occurring cancer. Because of this, the immune system of a healthy mouse can destroy FBL-3 cancer cells. I considered our experiments with FBL-3 an extension of the skin-graft work, with little direct relevance to an actual cancer therapy.

But FBL-3 *was* a cancer. The fact that we had advanced to the point of working with a cancer was itself encouraging. And what I intended was a strenuous test to find out whether T cells could be grown in IL-2 and work throughout an animal.

I assigned this project to Timothy Eberlein and asked Maury to help guide him. Tim arrived at NIH the same day Maury did but spent his first six months on the clinical service and did not come into my lab until January 1, 1980. He and Maury were opposites, worked side by side, and got along famously.

Tim's father was a factory foreman and Tim had attended the University of Pittsburgh on a football scholarship, a few years before they won the national championship. He went to medical school there, then became a resident at the Brigham. I am told football coaches tell players to "make something happen." That may be fairly typical of a surgeon's attitude. It certainly described Tim. He wanted action and results and he wanted them right now. Not all that big physically, still he was solid and had a physical presence. His mentality was that of a classic surgeon: aggressive, intense, competitive.

Tim was as green as anyone I ever accepted into the lab; his entire background in immunology consisted of two weeks in medical school. Maury taught him much: immunology, lab techniques, how to read a scientific paper. But he could not teach patience, and Tim's attitude toward the lab left little room for patience: "Just tell me what to do," he seemed to be saying, "and I'll do it." Not surprisingly, this left him open to frustration. He and Maury were an odd couple—Maury's reaction to failure was a quiet, rejuvenating walk; Tim pounded his fist fiercely against the desk, frustrated that he had nothing else to hit.

The FBL-3 model we began with had already been used by Alexander Fefer and his team in Seattle. They had shown that killer T cells could be generated by repeatedly immunizing normal black mice against the FBL-3 tumor. They had already taken T cells from these healthy, immunized black mice and given them directly—he had not grown them in culture—to other black mice suffering from the FBL-3 cancer. The T cells had cured the cancer.

I wanted to take Fefer's work several steps further by testing the ability of T cells grown in IL-2 to treat the cancer.

Fefer had by now also become interested in IL-2 and was doing the same thing. We were making progress when he published his results: T cells cultured in IL-2 and sensitized to FBL-3 cancers worked exactly as did T cells transferred directly from live, immunized animals.

My goal had never been simply to use Fefer's model. It had limitations and I was planning a new and more realistic tumor model. But Tim, competitive as he was, grew both angry and despondent. He thought his work was going nowhere.

The tedium of it began to overwhelm him. He was growing IL-2 in hundreds and hundreds of postcard-size plates; each plate had twenty-four separate wells, and he had to fill each well individually with a pipette the size of an elongated nose dropper. It was numbing to the mind, the forearm, and the thumb. Tim pounded his fist over every flask that got contaminated, every batch of IL-2 that did not work, every assay that gave an unexpected and meaningless result, every mouse that died accidentally—each one of these things destroyed days or weeks of work. I brought him into my office repeatedly, reassured him that this was the pace at which science moved, that he was doing nothing wrong, that in fact he was doing well, and he would leave ready to attack again.

Maury encouraged him also. Frequently he would suggest they get pizza and beer in the evening. They went to Shakey's, where they could have all they could eat for $5.99, and stayed for hours, eating, drinking beer, laughing, talking through the experiments. Maury had a gentle way of prodding, of communicating his own enthusiasm and perhaps his own frustrations. The next day they would come in rejuvenated.

Meanwhile I designed the tumor model I wanted. Fefer—we had so far done the same thing—had injected tumor cells into the abdomen, and then also injected the lymphocytes into the abdomen. But we needed to know whether the T cells cultured in IL-2 could kill cancer cells at distant sites.

I decided to inject the tumor cells into the footpad of the mice, wait until the cancer was well established and spread throughout the animal, and then inject the T cells into the tail vein, just as we had done in the skin-graft experiments. This would truly test whether the immune cells could travel and kill everywhere in the animal.

Tim began what was by now a familiar routine of working out the variables, such as how long to wait for the tumor to establish itself in the footpad and how many cells to inject. By now he could smell the end, smell the reward after all the frustration. This made him more intense than ever. His appointment was for two years. It was expiring and we were not finished. I offered him a third year. He leaped at the chance to stay.

Now he was rolling, setting up huge experiments, each one involving 150 to 200 animals, so many that we had to keep them at a contractor's building. And as we edged closer to the results we had predicted, as I opened the envelopes to break the code of each new experiment, he became more anxious and more determined to succeed.

Each experiment required an enormous expenditure of effort, yet the death of one mouse could conceivably ruin everything. Sometimes when the cells were injected into the mice, an animal asphyxiated. When this happened it seemed to become the focus of all of Tim's past frustrations. He could not tolerate it and once said, "I cannot express my emotion when—after spending months growing the cells and the whole day from 6:00 A.M. to 4:00 P.M. harvesting and preparing them, then finally injecting them—I have to watch the mouse seize and die."

I remember when one mouse had a seizure after a cell infusion, Tim ripped the plunger off the syringe, stuck one end in the animal's mouth and the other in his own, and gave mouth-to-mouth resuscitation to this small black mouse, trying to get it breathing again. He could not.

But if he became emotional—furious—over these events, he also became emotional watching a tumor, after treatment, begin to disappear. I became emotional, too.

In an experiment in late 1981, we achieved our first cure. Every untreated animal died within twenty-four days after injection of tumor cells. But with 50 million cultured and sensitized T cells, 80 percent of the treated animals—animals with large, established tumors as well as disseminated metastases—survived indefinitely. T cells had found and killed the FBL-3 cells everywhere in the animal.

We repeated the experiment. This time we cured 100 percent of the mice who received the sensitized T cells. All the controls again died.

We got this result again and again. We changed the variables to learn more about the killing mechanism in both the skin-graft and FBL-3 models and to explore every parameter, lowered the number of cells, confirmed specificity. And over and over we got the same results. Every control animal died. And most treated animals survived.

In both the skin graft and FBL-3 models, T cells cultured in IL-2 could work when injected into an animal.

And we observed one interesting complication. In our many experiments, we discovered that the T cells that killed best in test tubes did not kill best in an animal. Tests with irradiated killer cells were particularly interesting. Irradiated cells can function normally in many ways but they cannot divide and grow. In culture they killed target cells from the skin-graft donor. But irradiated cells had no effect at all in a living animal. These results suggested that something other than killing ability alone determined whether the treatment would work.

What did? We would have to address that question later.

For now it was more than enough that the second *if* was solved.

CHAPTER NINE

Magic and science have much in common.

Shortly after finishing my Ph.D. and returning to my residency, I contracted hepatitis. Able to do nothing but lie around for four months, I drove Alice crazy. She insisted that I find something to occupy myself and gave me a book on magic tricks. It enthralled me. I began to read more and more about the subject, mastered tricks of increasing complexity, and ultimately joined the International Brotherhood of Magicians.

One sees a magic trick and it seems incomprehensible, as if it just cannot be. Then, as one learns the principle behind the trick, one gets a flash of insight and it seems so obvious. In science, as in magic, if one can just learn the secret . . .

Answering the first two *ifs* was not a deep intellectual challenge. I had not known whether the answers would confirm or destroy my hypothesis, but I had known that an answer would be definitive. T cells either grew in IL-2 and maintained their killing ability or they did not. They either worked in a living animal or they did not.

Advancing the hypothesis further was different. Now we were dealing directly with cancer. And we were trying to find something that most immunologists believed did not exist. But as complex as the problem was, we were finally engaging the disease directly. And what we were doing could lead directly to treating patients.

In our previous experiments with the FBL-3 tumor, we had obtained immune cells by repeatedly immunizing a *normal* mouse with cancer cells. This would not be a feasible approach in humans.

The third *if* required us to find immune system cells *in a tumor-bearing animal—or a person with cancer*—that could recognize and attack the tumors, grow those cells in IL-2, and test their killing activity in culture. This was essential if we were ever to treat humans with cancer.

To do this we had to identify a natural immune response to cancer—one that was naturally occurring in an animal or a person with the disease—and isolate whatever element of the immune system was responding. I expected that this would be a T lymphocyte.

Where might I find such a T cell?

There were several logical places to search. One was the spleen, which is comprised mostly of lymphocytes. If anticancer lymphocytes existed, some would probably be present in the spleen.

Other scientists had already searched in the spleen for these lymphocytes. They had failed to find them. I had searched in the spleen myself, also unsuccessfully. This proved nothing. The spleen contained tens of millions of lymphocytes. It was possible that as few as a single one recognized cancer as foreign. Searching for this one sometimes made me think of screening an entire beach for a single, particular grain of sand.

I decided to focus my search in a location where a higher concentration of antitumor cells was likely to exist. My intuition told me that if the immune system was doing battle against cancer, then immune cells would most likely be found in the tumor itself. This is where I intended to look. Other scientists had also already looked in tumors for these cells and failed to find them. I thought we could do better.

I wanted to work with a tumor model similar to cancers that people develop. I chose a sarcoma induced by the laboratory chemical methylcholanthrene, or MCA, because I thought that MCA-caused cancers most closely resembled naturally occurring cancers in man. Key to this similarity is that MCA cancers are each unique. If ten different mice receive MCA, each resulting cancer will have slightly different properties. This is true even when all the mice belong to the same inbred strain. Similarly, all cancers in people are probably unique.

Once we induced several cancers, we kept them alive indefinitely, either by growing the cells in culture or transplanting them from animal to animal. We thus established several tumor cell lines by serially transplanting them in mice, and we numbered these cell lines. We began working with what we called the MCA-100 series—tumors called MCA-101, MCA-102, MCA-103, and so on.

One other thing we did was important. We did not transplant cancers indefinitely from animal to animal. If we had, the cancers would have inevitably changed and developed unnatural characteristics. Instead, we cryopreserved—froze at $-180°$ Celsius— cancer cells from the animals originally given MCA. We were constantly thawing these original cells and giving them to mice. That guaranteed that the cancer we studied resembled a naturally occurring wild one and not a mutated special-case situation.

We would use these tumors in our attempts to find immune cells in a mouse *bearing* a cancer that would attack the cancer. I expected this to be the most time-consuming of the five obstacles we faced. So, more than a year before Maury Rosenstein arrived, we began our efforts to overcome it. It was a gamble. All the effort would have been wasted if Maury and Tim had not succeeded. But it was the fastest way to achieve the goal. And Maury and Tim did succeed.

Ilana Yron is an Israeli scientist who had then just finished her Ph.D. and sent me her résumé. I was in Israel and interviewed her in the lobby of the Tel Aviv Hilton Hotel. She was an immunologist, very intelligent, and very alive to the world. I hired her. She joined the lab in July 1978, and I asked her to isolate lymphocytes infiltrating into MCA-100 series tumors, and to look for those lymphocytes that specifically recognize tumor.

In other experiments we had used a variety of different MCA-100 series tumors. All had acted similarly. Because of this, in Ilana's experiments we used only the MCA-102 cancer, a vicious one that grows very rapidly. We did not know it at the time but it turned out to be a critical choice, a choice that would consume our attention—and also delay other, more significant progress—for five years.

Ilana began by transplanting tumors into mice and after two weeks, when the tumors were large, surgically removing them. She then digested the tumors with enzymes to make single cell suspensions—in which all cells are dispersed throughout a liquid medium—and tried to separate out the lymphocytes. This was complex work. She then tested the lymphocytes for killing activity.

She spent six months doing this. The lymphocytes she did succeed in isolating—after enormous effort—did not recognize and kill the tumor.

This discouraged her. It wasn't only that the experiments were going poorly; I think working in tumor immunology disturbed her as well. The field was not considered part of the mainstream of immunology, and when she later left our lab she left this field as well. Perhaps another conflict was that I wanted her largely to describe phenomena, describe what cells were present and what their activities were. She wanted to do work at a more theoretical and analytical level. I felt what she wanted would not move me closer to my goal. At that point I felt we needed a broad view of what was occurring before we began to probe more deeply.

But Ilana's focus began to drift. She played the flute and seemed to devote more passion to it than her science. I believed her other activities were interfering with her science and told her so. She had to work harder. I told her of my belief that an investigator who begins a series of experiments without confidence often abandons them too quickly, instead of making them work. If her first approach proved unproductive, she would have to try others.

We talked about this and decided upon several alternative approaches. One was to grow lymphocytes we had isolated from a tumor in IL-2, even though we had no evidence that they attacked the tumor cells. The lymphocytes grew well. We decided to test their killing ability by mixing them with cells from the tumor. We obtained a startling result.

The lymphocytes grown in IL-2 killed the cancer cells.

The killing was weak but definite. We quickly set up a formal experiment that repeated the findings. Then Ilana added IL-2 to a mixture of tumor cells and lymphocytes. The tumor cells settled to the bottom and initially grew in a one-cell-thick carpet on the surface of the culture plate. A few days later Ilana noticed little islands appearing in the layer of tumor cells. The islands were clear. They seemed to be free of tumor.

Ilana examined the plate under the microscope. At the center of the clear islands were lymphocytes. Lymphocytes were killing tumor cells. She could see it! In our other experiments we could measure killing only with great difficulty in sensitive assays. This was happening under our eyes.

We immediately set up a larger experiment with several controls. One involved exposing the lymphocytes to a tumor different from the one from which they had been isolated. If our hypothesis was correct—that the lymphocytes had specifically recognized and killed the tumor cells—the cells from the second tumor would not be harmed.

The lymphocytes killed the control tumor cells, cells to which they had never been exposed before, cells they should not have recognized. We were puzzled and added other control tumors that should have been left unharmed. They, too, were killed.

This was an astonishing phenomenon. A basic tenet of immunology is that immune reactions are *specific*. Each lymphocyte should have only one specific target. But these lymphocytes cultured in IL-2 were killing *non*specifically. They killed every tumor target they encountered.

How was this occurring? What mechanism was at work?

We did not know.

In addition, the nonspecific killing was very weak. But the biggest issue remained the nonspecific nature of the killing. The nonspecific killing was so unexpected and puzzling that we wondered if the phenomenon was the result of some contaminant, rather than something real that we should explore and build upon.

We tried many other approaches to find killer cells that specifically attacked individual cancers. We could not find them.

What we did not know was that we were being blocked by extraordinarily bad luck. What we did know was that we were stymied.

While Ilana worked with murine cells, Michael Lotze followed along with human cells. Of all the people who have ever worked in my lab, Mike Lotze was among the two or three with the most talent and promise. He may also have been the most competitive. His grandfather was a physician and his wife, Joan, was a physician. His father-in-law, A. McGee Harvey, had been a nationally prominent chief of medicine at Johns Hopkins, and his mother-in-law and one sister-in-law were also physicians.

There was a hunger in Mike to learn, to help, but also to achieve and be recognized for his achievement. He was one of those people who needed to take part in the action. If someone else's work was going well, he wanted to be part of it. And this aggressiveness offended some of his colleagues. Once we had a discussion about whether it was worth being in the public domain—whether it was worth being famous. He told me he thought it was, that maybe it would inspire some child, that every generation needed heroes. Mike wanted to be a hero.

He arrived a month before Ilana but began on the clinical service. When his time to rotate into the lab arrived, he asked to work directly with me, but for several weeks I vacillated between choosing him and someone else. I finally chose Mike because I thought he would work harder. In retrospect, I am surprised at my failure to perceive his ability more clearly.

Some investigators find uncertainty difficult to accept; before proceeding on anything new, they read every article written on the subject. They begin experiments timidly and, needing the comfort of certainty, hesitate to build on something they do not understand fully. They do not fully appreciate that all science begins with doubt. Wanting everything perfect can paralyze them, and progress for them comes slowly, if at all.

Others begin work on the authority of their superiors. Not confident of their own ideas, they take advice too readily. When encountering obstacles, they always seek the guidance of others and resist trying new things. They can do good science, but rarely do they generate much creativity.

And a rare few people react to a problem or a suggestion with excitement; before the conversation ends they are planning experiments. They dive in, learn as they proceed, attack and attack. They are driven either by the particular goal or by their love for the process of science itself. They can survive on the edge, and out on the edge is where real scientific work is done. Science isn't found in books. It's in the laboratory or in nature. I feel, as Emerson wrote, "Books are for a scholar's idle times. When he can read God directly, the hour is too precious to be wasted in other men's transcripts of their readings."

Mike Lotze devoured projects in a way few people in my group have ever done. He loved the lab and on occasion slept in the wards so he could watch data come off counters in the middle of the night. I recall when his wife was about to have a baby. Her water broke at 2:00 A.M. and he left immediately for the lab to tend all his cultures because, as he later said, he knew he would be tied up for some time. Then he returned home and took his wife to the hospital in Baltimore.

Our own relationship was unique. We spent inordinate amounts of time together. Others in the lab seemed to grow jealous. Mike did demand attention from me. But he was generating enormous amounts of data while I often had to pull results out of others.

He began working on several projects, doing with human cells what others had already done in mice. Soon he caught up and began the search for human immune system cells that would kill cancer cells.

Mike experimented with lymphocytes from blood and tumors taken from cancer patients in the hospital. He started to isolate and grow these lymphocytes in IL-2. They killed tumor cells.

This *was* the same phenomenon Ilana had seen.

Mike, like Ilana, wanted to abandon work with these nonspecific killers. Nothing in immunology functioned as they did. He was worried that no papers written about the cells would be published. Both Mike and Ilana, and most others in the lab, believed the killing was an unnatural artifact induced by either an unknown contaminant or some experimental procedure.

I had no explanation for the phenomenon, but the fact that we had seen it in both human and murine cells made me think it was a real event, not an artifact, not the result of an experimental flaw. Yet these strange cells were not what I had been looking for and seemed almost to stand in the way of finding more powerful *specific* killers of cancer cells.

At the same time, in a technical sense we had solved the third *if*.

We had found immune cells in a tumor-bearing animal that attacked the animal's cancer.

And we had found immune cells in people with cancer that killed their cancer cells.

This thought overpowered me: I could not bear the idea that we had cells that could kill a human cancer, even if only weakly in a test tube, and not use them. I wanted to give these cells to patients, I wanted to do it right now, and I wanted to do it no matter what.

My desire to seek permission for an immediate clinical trial to treat patients with these nonspecific killer cells raised a complex ethical issue in my own mind. Did we know enough to justify the risks to the patient?

In war, one can knowingly sacrifice a company to save a battalion, or a battalion to save a division, or an army to save a nation. One makes judgments based on one's view of the forest, not the trees. Public policy also usually seeks the greatest good for the greatest number.

Clinical medicine is different. In medicine, the best interests of the individual patient being treated must at all times take precedence over all other considerations. In medicine, it would be unethical to sacrifice one individual even to save millions in the future. In medicine, an ethical doctor must ignore the forest and focus solely on one tree at a time.

Clinical research similarly differs from basic research. In basic research one studies a disease. In clinical research one studies a patient with a disease. One must weigh possible benefits against possible risks in each individual case.

But when trying new therapies one does not clearly know either the risks or the benefits. A tension can exist between the patient's best interest and the investigator's desire to learn by attempting something new. If I needed to know the answer to a question to help others—and I did—did this need cloud my judgment?

I did not fool myself. I knew that it was extremely unlikely that giving a patient these cells would cause his or her cancer to regress. Even in the pig lymphocyte experiments, we had more reason to believe the therapy might succeed than we did now; Symes, the English scientist, had at least claimed positive results. Yet we knew too little to dismiss out of hand the possibility that it could help a patient. I felt, or perhaps just hoped, that there was a chance it could work. Perhaps treatment with these cells might stimulate some kind of chain reaction among other immune system cells in the body. Perhaps in trying this, unexpected things would happen that would open doors for us to help other patients. I kept thinking of Franny Moore's comment that chance favors the prepared mind only when the mind is at work.

And if the likely benefits were small, we would be treating terminally ill patients who had exhausted all alternative therapies. I judged the risks to them also to be small. True, IL-2-grown lymphocytes had never been given to patients before and unknown risks might exist. But animals given comparable numbers of cells grown in IL-2 had had no problems. And we had already given huge numbers of pig lymphocytes to people without ill effects.

I sought permission from the clinical research committee for patient trials and presented my reasoning, along with an explicit scientific goal we expected to achieve.

I felt it was essential to ask a well-defined question even if the patients were not helped. It was the only guarantee we would learn something. We intended to study the trafficking of the lymphocytes. We would label them with a radioactive isotope (after some experimentation we settled on indium-111), perform nuclear scans, and examine where in the body the cells went. These studies could bring us important information for future patients. We had already performed such work in mice.

The clinical protocol was approved.

The patients to whom I offered this therapy had no other treatment options. I worried that we might unrealistically raise their hopes only to destroy them again. In a way, the detailed informed-consent agreements that the patients read and we discussed eased these concerns. I told them we had no reason to believe the therapy would work. We had no animal models that showed it would work. We did not know what would happen to the cells once they entered the body, so there was some risk. We feared that because these IL-2-grown cells were so much larger than normal lymphocytes, they might get clogged in the lungs.

The only positive thing I could say was that in a test tube their lymphocytes killed their tumors.

Nelson Edwards was a fifty-three-year-old man, an alcoholic with severe cirrhosis of his liver. He was separated from his wife. We admitted him to the hospital on April 3, 1979, with a large mass, a sarcoma, in his upper thigh. Because of the size of his tumor, local excision was impossible. I recommended a hemi-pelvectomy—an amputation at the hip. He was a hunter who liked to get outdoors and declined, explaining, "I want to be able to play with my grandchildren physically."

A month later Mr. Edwards changed his mind. We amputated his leg in May. But in a December follow-up visit we discovered aggressive, rapidly growing tumors in both lungs, a mass in his neck, and a bony metastasis in his jaw, which was very painful.

He received radiation therapy for the pain, but we could not give him chemotherapy. It would have been too dangerous because of his liver disease.

I explained what we wanted to do with lymphocytes. He agreed to try it. He had nothing else. We removed lymphocytes from his blood and grew them for four weeks in IL-2. On January 29, 1980, at 9:20 A.M., we gave him 150 million cells labeled with indium-111.

We scanned him using a gamma camera to detect radioactivity in his body after the infusion of cells at two hours, six hours, twenty-four hours, and nine days. At first the cells accumulated in the lung, which we had feared, but over a four-hour period most went to the spleen and liver.

To our disappointment, they did not accumulate at tumor sites at all.

A month later his tumors had grown. After a few more months he died.

The findings in our studies were consistent for the first three patients. No tumors responded and all the patients ultimately died of progressive cancer. There was not even a hint of any beneficial effect.

A single gram of tumor contains one billion cells. The patients had kilogram tumor burdens—trillions of tumor cells. In culture we had found that it required dozens of the nonspecific killer lymphocytes to kill a single tumor cell, and we were only giving the patients 150 million lymphocytes.

Watching Mr. Edwards and the other two patients die killed my private hope that somehow the lymphocytes would stimulate other immune system cells to respond to the cancer. That had not happened. Now I knew this effort could not work. It was futile.

I had to stop. We had solved the third *if*. We had found immune cells in cancer patients that recognized and destroyed their cancer cells in a test tube. But I had tried to jump too far ahead. Until we better understood what was happening, we would treat no more patients. We had to go back to the lab.

PART THREE

PURSUIT

CHAPTER TEN

The beginning of July marks a changing of seasons for me. Fellows and surgical residents whom I have worked with for two or three years and come to know intimately leave to continue their training or join university faculties or go into practice. A new group of fellows arrives. They bring freshness to the lab, a new eagerness and vitality, but training them in our research and techniques can disrupt the flow of the work.

On July 1, 1980, John Strausser went back to Boston to finish his residency. Ilana Yron accepted another postdoctoral fellowship in New York. Mike Lotze went to Strong Memorial Hospital in Rochester, New York, to finish his residency, although I hoped to bring him back later. Maury Rosenstein and Tim Eberlein remained, and arriving in my lab were Elizabeth Grimm, a Ph.D. scientist, Amitabha Mazumder, Ben Kim, and, later, John Donohue, all M.D.s. Only Liz Grimm had any laboratory background.

The influx of new people changed my role somewhat. I had an increasing number of investigators in my own lab, and responsibilities as chief of the Surgery Branch continued to weigh upon me. To help handle administrative details, I leaned more and more on Alan Baker. We had been residents together at the Brigham, and I had asked him to come with me to NCI. We started the same day. Al is my friend, and one of the most solid, logic-driven, and honest people I have ever known. If he says he will do something, it is done. He is also an obsessive clinician who misses nothing and attends to every detail; our fellows nominated him for, and he won, an NIH award for outstanding clinical teaching. As the years went on, he took on a heavier and heavier clinical and administrative load for me, for example, sitting in for me on the Surgical Administrative Committee, which oversees the O.R. I trust him both to take care of things on his own and to keep me informed if there is something I need to know.

Even with his and others' help, I had to reorganize my time. As my own lab expanded, as more and more people in it simultaneously pursued different questions, as our work stopped moving in a straight line and broadened and deepened and branched out, people began to proceed down separate tracks. Although I continued to perform experiments personally with Sue Schwarz and Paul Spiess, I also began spending more time as an adviser, insuring that those tracks continued in the right direction.

I always gave everyone a specific area of responsibility. Some lab chiefs operate differently; they try to generate creative tensions by having fellows or postdocs work on the same thing. I do not see science as a competition, and having independent responsibilities encourages colleagues to hope for one another's success. Indeed, for our project to succeed each individual had to succeed. Pressure came not from any artificial competition; it came from knowing the patients who lay a few steps down the corridor from the lab, dying of cancer in our ward.

While we continued to search for a definitive solution to the third *if*—the strange, nonspecific killer cells we had found continued to puzzle and dissatisfy us—other people worked on other questions. What happened to T cells when they entered the body? Which cell subpopulations were responsible for rejecting the skin grafts and killing FBL-3 cells? What were the implications for activity against cancer? What were the characteristics of the nonspecific killer cells we had found? Could they be made powerful enough to use in therapy? Were there other ways to generate nonspecific killers that did not require IL-2? What happened to IL-2 in vivo?

We needed to know . . . *everything*.

Later, if everything proceeded as I hoped, I intended to bring all those tracks together in the effort to destroy a growing cancer in a patient. The next moment that we seemed to take a significant step forward, I intended to treat patients again.

One of the first things we needed to do was understand more about the functioning of T cells. Ben Kim spent his years in my lab working on one thing: trying to find out what kind of T cell worked best in vivo and how. To study this he cloned individual T cells—from a single parent cell he grew a population of millions of identical daughter cells—and searched for the ones most effective in destroying foreign skin grafts. His results were unexpected.

He confirmed what earlier experiments by Maury had suggested: that killing ability in culture did not correlate with killing ability in an animal. Only lymphocytes that in culture could both kill and proliferate in response to antigen speeded the rejection of grafts.

IL-2 was already important to us. The fact that it could turn lymphocytes into nonspecific killers added to its importance and intensified my interest in it. Ben Kim's findings elevated its significance even higher.

IL-2 made lymphocytes grow. If only cells that could grow inside an animal could work, then giving IL-2 to animals—and ultimately patients—could be vital in developing effective therapies. IL-2 could be as important to immunotherapy as immune system cells themselves.

I now knew I would give IL-2 to animals—and, depending on the results, to patients. In my mind, I designed what I called "the Cinderella experiment," a fairy-tale experiment in which we would give animals large numbers of immune lymphocytes that could kill cancer along with huge amounts of IL-2. If the IL-2 kept those killer cells alive and growing, growing until they flooded every artery, patrolled every capillary, infiltrated every organ, and sought out every cancer cell in the body . . . what would happen then?

A fairy-tale aspect of the experiment involved the scarcity of IL-2. For now we had only enough IL-2 to grow cells in culture.

Giving it to animals would certainly require vastly greater quantities. Also, our IL-2 was not pure—we had removed the lectin from the supe but the IL-2 remained diluted in it. Other contaminants were also present. And it took great effort to get what little supplies we had.

Still, I began to prepare for using IL-2 in vivo by learning more about it. My first question was how long after injection it survived in an animal's bloodstream. Blood moves rapidly through an animal. In man, the circulation time is approximately fourteen seconds. That means that every blood cell in the body passes through the lungs, the heart, arteries and veins in other parts of the body, and back into the heart every fourteen seconds. In mice, blood cells pass through the circulatory system even faster.

I performed the first experiments myself to find IL-2's survival time in murine circulatory systems, then asked John Donohue to continue the work. We found that mice eliminated IL-2 very rapidly; given intravenously, IL-2 had a half-life of 3.7 minutes, meaning that the body eliminated half of it in that time.

This was not good news. It meant that only repeated dosages of IL-2 would have any effect in vivo. We would need huge quantities to explore its potential. People would also very likely eliminate IL-2 quickly. If so, any human therapy involving IL-2 would also require enormous amounts.

How could we ever get such quantities?

Already the lab was purchasing IL-2 supe from a contractor who used the procedures we had developed. Even so, we could get only tiny amounts. In the back of my mind was the hope that genetic engineering and the biotechnology industry might provide the answer to the supply problem, but I had no idea whether that answer would come in two years or twenty years.

In the meantime, there had to be either a substitute for IL-2 or better sources of it. We began looking for both.

The search for new sources of IL-2 began. The search for immune cells in people that *specifically* destroy their cancers continued. The nonspecific killers we had found seemed too weak to work in a therapy. If we were ever to treat patients, we had to do better.

Liz Grimm started her work in the lab searching for such specific cells. Scientists in Sweden and England reported that they had generated these specific killer T cells by mixing, in vitro, lymphocytes and cancer cells from the same patient. They reported that they got specificity—cells that recognized the patient's cancer cells but nothing else.

Good science must be reproducible. We could not reproduce these results. For six months Liz tried and failed. When she added IL-2 all she got was the same nonspecific killers we had observed before. The reported results were either flawed or the product of a set of circumstances unique to their laboratory.

Her failures were disheartening to her. She is a strong-willed feminist and highly competitive, yet she thought of quitting the project. Perhaps her very competitiveness made her so distraught. She did not quit, but she could not find a way past this obstacle; she seemed unable to avoid creating these nonspecific killers. My ideas worked no better than hers. Wherever we turned, whatever we tried, we ran into a wall.

Not only did we consider these nonspecific killers too weak to be useful, but we also believed they were interfering with our finding specific killer T lymphocytes. Finally we decided that if we were ever to get past these cells we would have to understand them better. So Liz began full-time studies to characterize them. Over a period of more than a year she examined these cells in exquisite detail.

It was a turning point.

Liz Grimm's characterization of these cells was absolutely first-rate science. She explored the best ways to generate them, discovered their precursors, and defined their capabilities. The more we learned about them, the more interested we became in them.

Liz realized they were a class of lymphocytes never previously recognized. She wanted to give them a name. We called them lymphokine-activated killer cells, or LAK cells. Lymphokines are proteins secreted by lymphocytes that carry messages between them; IL-2 is a lymphokine.

We had uncovered a whole new area of immunology. In retrospect, I am surprised how long it took us to see the importance of the phenomenon. Our first paper on LAK cells became a "citation classic," a name given to a handful of papers most cited by other scientists.

When we began studying LAK cells, we considered them unwanted interlopers; when we finished, we viewed them as if we were proud and possessive parents.

Now, in light of our inability to find more specific killers, we began thinking about how we might use them—in patients. But we were still hamstrung by a lack of IL-2. It was like some glass barrier that imprisoned us. We could see through it, see the experiments we wanted to perform just on the other side of the glass, but we could not penetrate it.

I asked Amitabha Mazumder, a new fellow, to look for ways to generate killer cells without IL-2. For once a project turned out to be easier than expected. Soon we were generating nonspecific human killer cells by culturing human lymphocytes with lectin alone. (This probably occurred because the lymphocytes themselves, stimulated by the lectin, produced some IL-2.) The lectin we used for this was phytohemagglutinin, which comes from plants. Unlike IL-2, it was readily available in bulk.

For the first time we could produce large numbers of killer cells, cells that killed cancers.

Later studies showed that these cells performed exactly as LAK cells did. Like LAK cells, they were far from perfect. They killed weakly. But they did kill. If their killing fitted no paradigm of immunology, if some scientists even in my own lab still considered them an artificial creation of our experimental system, we had observed this killing and had faith in our observations.

I began to wonder about generating huge numbers of lectin-activated killer cells from a patient with cancer. The first three cancer patients who had received IL-2-activated killer cells had gotten a minuscule quantity of cells. We had not had enough IL-2 to generate more. Now using lectin, we could give perhaps a hundred times as many killer cells as the earlier patients had received. Could these cells destroy a patient's cancer? The question itself compelled me to act.

Almost immediately I wanted to give lectin-activated killer cells to patients.

Amitabha's experiments were conducted in late 1980 and January and February of 1981. In March I applied to the clinical research committee of NCI for permission to conduct clinical trials with these cells.

Risk to the patients did exist. Some of the techniques we intended to employ were not yet fully understood, and the lectin-activated killers were much larger than normal lymphocytes and also clumped more. We feared they could clog the lungs and cause an infarction. This would be a life-threatening complication.

And we had no animal models to justify our request. There was a reason for this lack of animal data: Only with IL-2—not with lectin—could we generate killer cells in the one mouse strain in which we had generated all our tumors. If we wanted to run experiments with these lectin-activated cells in mice we would have to start everything—including growing new cancers—from scratch. This could delay us a year or more.

I did not want to wait. Our patients could not wait.

And there were good reasons to proceed. On the basis of our experience with the pig lymphocytes and the earlier killer-cell infusions, I considered the risk to the patients reasonable. Also, a clinical trial could generate much practical information—such as how to handle a very large number of a patient's cells—that we would need to know before designing an effective therapy, assuming we ever did find more potent killer cells. Finally, perhaps my determination to go ahead reflected Schopenhauer's observation that one sign of man's desperation is the alacrity with which he grasps hope. I did have hope. I thought the cells might just work.

On May 11, 1981, Bruce Chabner, the associate director of the

Clinical Oncology Program of NCI, approved the protocol. I had been awaiting word anxiously and had already discussed the treatment with our first patient. The day Chabner approved the experiment, we admitted our first patient to the hospital for treatment.

Amanda Pritchard was from Newport, Rhode Island, and had first come to NIH two years earlier, a month before she was to be married. She was then twenty years old and had a mass in her thigh. A surgeon at her local hospital excised it; it was a grade 3 synovial cell sarcoma, one of the most vicious cancers. When cutting out a tumor, the surgeon always tries to cut around it; if one cuts across or punctures a tumor, cancer cells can leak into the local area and begin to grow at new sites. In Amanda's case, the tumor was intimately wrapped around critical blood vessels; to avoid damaging the blood vessels, the surgeon had to enter the tumor. It spilled throughout the wound. He referred Amanda to us.

A surgical fellow and I reoperated, cleaned the area, and recommended radiation and chemotherapy as additional treatment. Amanda accepted radiation but refused chemotherapy. She did not want to lose her hair before her wedding.

She was exceptionally attractive, in fact beautiful, but her decision had nothing to do with a superficial concern about her appearance. Her decision was a profound one. She, her fiancé, and I talked over the diagnosis and its implications in detail. Her fiancé gave her total support. I remember vividly the dignity with which she carried herself. She told me, "I prefer a shortened life in which I can do what I enjoy, compared to a longer life which is miserable." At the same time she said, "This cancer is going to get me."

She was married on July 21, 1979. A year and a half later X rays revealed that the cancer had spread to her lungs. We performed an immediate thoracotomy and removed all of her lung tumors, but there were many. She accepted chemotherapy. Her husband wanted her to. But on her next follow-up, in early May, more tumors had returned in both lungs.

I spoke in general with her about the experiment with killer

136

cells. She was interested. On the same day we received approval to proceed, I told her about it in detail. One issue we discussed was leukopheresis, one of several techniques we needed to perfect if we were ever to treat patients successfully. In pheresis, which had been developed largely at NIH, a patient's blood is diverted to circulate through a machine and then returned to the body. The machine separates lymphocytes and platelets from red blood cells and plasma, the liquid part of the blood. We would then take these lymphocytes and expose them to the lectin for two days, and then infuse them into the patient's bloodstream.

We planned to perform as many as fifteen phereses over a period of a few weeks. Other researchers were also trying repeated, multiple phereses for patients suffering from autoimmune diseases, including rheumatoid arthritis. (In these diseases lymphocytes attack the body's own cells. Researchers reasoned that removing lymphocytes would help victims of these diseases.) But the risks of repeated phereses were still unclear. No one knew if cancer patients could tolerate them.

But there was no alternative treatment. She wanted to enter the protocol.

The same day Amanda Pritchard was admitted we pheresed her and removed large numbers of lymphocytes. Her husband was at her side every instant. Two days later, on May 13, I placed her in the Intensive Care Unit to reinfuse her cells. If the cells were going to clog the lungs and cause an embolism, which could kill her, we needed to be prepared to deal with it.

The cells were also labeled radioactively so we could track them. An electrocardiogram monitored her heartbeat, and the ICU nurses, Amitabha, and I stood at the foot of her bed in case any problems occurred during the cell infusion.

At first we infused a test dose of 100,000 cells. She did not react at all. Then, slowly, over an hour, we dripped ten billion of her cells into her veins.

She developed a severe headache, chills, and shaking, and her temperature spiked to 39° Celsius—103° Fahrenheit. Her lung function decreased. The cells were trapped in her lungs. We grew anxious.

Then she stabilized. The next day the side effects dissipated. We repeated the cycle of pheresis and infusion nine times, and she received 72 billion cells over three weeks. Six weeks later she returned for evaluation.

Her tumors were growing.

We performed another thoracotomy to remove her lung tumors surgically. She had too many tumors to remove. There was a heavy silence in the operating room and a feeling of desperate and frustrating impotence as the wound was closed, leaving the cancer within.

Amanda Pritchard stayed with NCI and endured one after another experimental chemotherapy regimen. She endured that which she had earlier decided not to endure, and she died young. I often think of her.

We treated nine more patients. I recall one man, Tom Showard, a Vietnam veteran who believed Agent Orange had caused his cancer. One arm had been amputated. I remember with pain sitting with him in a room in our third-floor clinic and telling him that his lung tumors were growing, that the treatment had not worked. We talked for a while and he said, "You know one thing that really bothers me? I get angry at my kids for no reason. It's not fair to them."

I got to know all ten patients well. All ten died. But we did not stop. Instead we changed the protocol and added cyclophosphamide, a chemotherapeutic agent, and modified the culture conditions.

Slowly, at the rate of barely one person a month, Amitabha and I continued to treat patients. We treated twenty-one patients with lectin-activated cells. None showed any indication of having benefited from the therapy, and all died of their cancers.

I had a difficult time dealing with their deaths. Failures in lab experiments were discouraging but I could always make a change and try again. Failures in these clinical trials yielded no second chances for the patients. This thought, although rarely expressed, was constantly in my mind as I spoke with the patients and their families. Time was running out for them. Patients place extraordinary trust in NIH doctors; they think that, enveloped as we are with science, we can cure anyone. I felt I could cure no one.

I felt guilty leaving these patients in the hospital and going home. How could I justify playing catch or checkers with my daughters, then ten and eight years old, while Amanda or Tom or the others, trusting in my ability to cure them, were struggling with both their cancers and the pain of the treatment? I tried to separate my family life from the hospital and thought that by staying longer hours I could leave this pain behind when I went home. And I spent more and more hours working.

Even so I never could leave it all behind. Years later, when my oldest daughter, Beth, was applying to colleges, I realized just how much I had brought home, and I wondered what impact all the failures had had on my own family. I thought this when Beth showed me an autobiographical essay she had written for one of her applications. She began with a statement that jolted me when I read it: "My father is a cancer surgeon and a research scientist. For as long as I can remember, discussions at our home have dealt as much with cancer and death as they have with the weather and the Washington Redskins."

CHAPTER ELEVEN

Twice now we had tried to leapfrog ahead and apply our laboratory findings instantly to patients. Twice we had failed. It was apparent that to succeed—if success was possible at all—we would have to follow the step-by-step path I had laid out earlier.

The answer had to be in the laboratory. I thought it might be IL-2, and I had to have it.

I had become more and more intrigued with IL-2, and it became more and more the focus of our experiments as I started exploring the effect IL-2 itself had on cancer.

And although we continued to look for immune cells that specifically killed a cancer, we accepted the nonspecific killer cells as a solution to the third *if*. They did kill cancer cells in culture. Now we wanted to find out whether these cells could overcome the fourth *if*. Could they kill cancer cells in an animal?

If the answer was yes, perhaps we could devise a way to successfully treat cancer patients with them.

Amitabha began a series of experiments using IL-2-activated killer cells against cancer in mice. In our patients we had seen no results from killer cells, but we could adjust a mouse model in ways impossible with patients. We could obviously test dangerous dosages in mice more easily than in patients, for example, and we could also use LAK cells against very small tumors. Our patients all had advanced cancer and heavy tumor burdens. It was possible that the cells might have no measurable effect on advanced cancer, but could still slow the growth of, or even cure, a smaller and less established tumor. If so, we needed to find out.

We began by testing LAK cells against MCA-102 tumors, a particularly vicious sarcoma. In one of Amitabha's first experiments, treated animals did better than control animals. The differences were not dramatic but they were real.

Amitabha was directly involved in the care of the patients receiving killer cells. He felt the same urgency to find a way to help them as I. He was grimly and determinedly enthusiastic.

But Amitabha could not repeat the results. He tried the experiment over and over without success. We did not understand why the treatment had worked once but would not again, and, try as he might, he could not identify the factor or factors responsible. It was possible that chance had accounted for the results.

So we started over and chose a new model. Instead of using the MCA-102 tumor, we decided to use an old cancer cell line dubbed "B16." In general I disliked using the B16 tumor line because it had existed in culture for decades and no longer resembled a naturally occurring cancer. Very likely it had developed qualities that made it a much easier target for immune system cells than a wild cancer. So I distrusted results obtained with it.

Still, we were trying to test a principle, and B16 was more akin to a wild cancer than a skin graft was. If we could get the model working with B16, we could then try to apply what we learned to the tougher MCA line—and, I hoped, to patients.

Amitabha quickly and repeatedly showed that the LAK cells could kill the B16 tumor in an animal. Seeing the results gave me a sudden lift. This was the first time we had seen reproducible decreases in tumors. But when we again used LAK cells in the more realistic MCA tumor model, we still could not measure any benefits.

Had we observed something real that we could build upon? Or had we only manipulated nature into yielding an artificial and misleading result?

While Amitabha studied LAK cells, Paul Spiess and I began focusing directly on IL-2. I had become enthralled with the idea of making cancer-killing cells grow inside a living animal.

Since IL-2 was the key to cell growth in culture, it made sense that it could also make anticancer cells grow in vivo. And the more we studied IL-2, the more impressed I became with its promise, and the more I felt we needed it.

I was not alone. By now IL-2 was drawing attention and creating excitement around the world, at least partly because of our work, much of which had by now become known; we had already published about a dozen papers on it.

But no one had solved the supply problem. Scientists had found several relatively high-producing cell lines. One high-producing human cell line was called Jurkat, named after the patient from whom the cells came. Steve Gillis from Dartmouth had discovered how to manipulate Jurkat cells into churning out relatively large quantities of human IL-2. Also, John Farrar at another NIH lab was using a high-producing mouse cell line, named the EL-4 line.

I spoke with John and he supplied me with some EL-4 cells. On August 26, 1981, Paul Spiess began cloning them to find the highest-producing single cell of the entire EL-4 line. This required a few months but when he finished we no longer had to kill mice to supply IL-2. We could grow it from our clones—billions of daughter cells descended from this one cell. Soon we had huge vats of EL-4 cultures growing.

This still did not solve the supply problem, but it did provide us with enough IL-2 to explore its potency. First we had to purify it—until now we had only eliminated the lectin. Paul and I spent weeks applying techniques I had learned studying proteins in graduate school. Finally we had a fairly pure protein. And I was anxious to test its power.

On November 17, 1981, in Paul's 398th experiment in my lab, we made our first attempt to treat tumors—and they were large tumors—with IL-2 alone, inside an animal. We made a huge batch of IL-2, approximately eight liters, and concentrated it eighty-fold to less than 100 milliliters.

This was barely enough to conduct an experiment. We could treat only two mice. Two control animals would get a saline solution. But if something is really impressive, even a tiny experiment can show important results.

Paul remembers the experiment well: "I wanted to inject them every four hours, so I took the mice home to inject them at night. I put them in the hall. I found out mice are nocturnal animals. They were very loud. It's amazing how much noise a few mice in a cage can make. My mother said, 'Well, they can't stay here.' On the way back to the lab it was very cold and the water bottle broke in the cage. The mice got wet. One died. That meant there was only one control. The experiment was ruined. But the tumors in the IL-2 group did shrink.''

The tumors did not shrink much, and all the mice eventually died of cancer. But tumors do not shrink by themselves. I was more anxious than ever to proceed. After all the years of frustration, we could sense we were on to something. We could taste it. We filled the lab with vats of cells producing IL-2, jammed them into every inch of incubator space. Where there weren't vats, there were flasks. We performed dozens of experiments. The mice, treated and untreated, continued to die. Results continued to be marginal.

But it was clear the IL-2 was doing something.

In autopsies on the mice, Elaine Jaffe, an NIH pathologist and an expert in lymphoid tissues, and I evaluated the mice that had received IL-2. We noted dramatic changes in the tissues of these animals. IL-2 was definitely having an effect.

Paul and I continued our efforts to make purer IL-2. We had used an eighty-fold concentration in our November 1981 experiment. By July 1982, we achieved a 1,000-fold concentration. With it we saw small—but consistent and real—decreases in tumors. A graph comparing treated and untreated mice was dramatic: The plot of the line showing tumors in untreated mice angled sharply up. For treated mice it went down—for a while.

We were still frustrated by the lack of IL-2; we did not have enough to give it in large doses. But on August 2, 1982, we tested its potency by injecting three groups of mice with IL-2 in different dilutions. Tumors in mice receiving the highest concentration of IL-2 remained stable; the cancer did not grow. In a 1:2 dilution, tumors were also stable. In a 1:4 dilution, tumor growth showed no difference from the control.

I had learned all I was going to from this series of experiments and stopped them. I asked Paul to refocus his attention on anti-cancer immune system cells.

But the experiments convinced me that the amount of IL-2 was crucial, and they also convinced me that IL-2 alone could have an effect on tumors. I now believed that if we could only give enough IL-2—if we could get enough—we could have an impact on cancer.

Every morning now I came into work excited, but also frustrated. Every night I talked about the work with Alice. Often we would take long walks around the block and I would go over the results of an experiment I had learned that day, what they meant, where we might head with them. And I was eager to get on with it. At the same time I felt as if there was a powerful machine at my disposal, that its enormous engine sat ready to roar, but that I could not find the key to it. I knew what the key was—huge quantities of high-quality IL-2—but I could not find it. Somewhere in the lab this key was hidden.

The different tracks down which our work had been going were beginning to converge. That only made our need for IL-2 more urgent, and made my frustration over the lack of it more intense.

We needed IL-2. The need was almost a physical, tangible one. But how could we get it? Where would we find it?

CHAPTER TWELVE

I had always considered Mike Lotze an exceptional young scientist and was eager to have him return to NCI. As he was finishing his surgical residency, I offered him a post as a senior investigator, along with his own lab and resources, although under my overall direction. Strong Memorial Hospital at the University of Rochester wanted him to stay on and offered him a position as head of their surgical oncology unit.

Despite the closeness of our relationship—or perhaps because of it—he was ambivalent about returning. I think much of his ambivalence came from his desire to establish himself as an independent scientist, and from a fear that if he returned to my lab people would not see him as his own man.

He rejected my offer and accepted the hospital's.

I offered the senior investigator post to Fred Chang, who accepted, did excellent work with me for five years, and left to become chief of surgical oncology at the University of Michigan. Meanwhile Mike's ambivalence intensified. He later said that one bleak day in Rochester he grew depressed and worried about finding a way to fund his research. He called the person at NCI who headed the grant program in his field and asked for an off-the-record, real-world evaluation of his chances of getting major grants. (Less than one-third of NIH's budget is spent in Bethesda; the rest funds research at universities around the country.) He was told that most of the money went to big, established labs. He did not want to have to fight for money. He wanted to do research. One of the greatest boons researchers at NIH enjoy is that they do not have to write grant proposals, which can easily take one-third of an investigator's time. Mike called me.

"Will you take me back?" he asked.

"Are you kidding?" I answered. "Of course."

The University of Rochester was upset enough that it demanded he repay $2,000 he had used to hire a technician. I was thrilled to have Mike return but the position I had first offered him was now filled. July 1, 1982, Mike came back into makeshift space.

In ways besides the location of his desk, he seemed almost as if he could not find his place. Once he said, "Most scientists live with doubt and worry at all times."

That comment is true, but with him it seemed to have a special meaning. When he was first in the lab, our relationship had been clear: I was mentor and he learned. Now it was more ambiguous. He had always been aggressive and competitive; now he became more so. We remained close yet he seemed to compete with me, too, as if he wanted to *be* me. He elbowed his way into other people's work, particularly the work with LAK cells, which Liz Grimm had taken over from him when he left. And she was almost as competitive as he.

At the same time nothing had happened to Mike's talent. It remained extraordinary. Generally when people come into the lab I give them small pieces of a task, but Mike was returning as a senior investigator. He needed something big enough to build an entire body of work around, and he had the ability to do large things. So I asked Mike to do something that was large. I told him, "I want you to purify IL-2 for clinical trials."

This was a difficult, frustrating project. It was also extraordinarily important.

Giving IL-2 to patients was our goal. Getting enough IL-2 for this seemed just short of impossible. We could barely make enough murine IL-2 to run the most preliminary experiments in mice. Treating patients would require quantities hundreds of times larger.

First Mike tried to get it from a gibbon monkey cell line, which makes IL-2 continuously (monkey IL-2 interacts with human and murine T cells, as well as with monkey cells). He spent months on it but generated only tiny amounts. It was becoming apparent that our lab would have to devote immense resources—resources I might not be able to get—to making IL-2.

Meanwhile Richard Robb at Du Pont published excellent work on IL-2 receptors on immune cells. In the course of his studies, he had purified human IL-2 from the Jurkat cell line; although he had generated only infinitesimal quantities of it, this IL-2 was considerably purer than the 1,000-fold concentration Paul Spiess and I had obtained from mice.

If Du Pont would supply us with pure human IL-2, our problem might be solved. Mike and I decided to try to convince Du Pont to do this.

Mike called Robb, who was intrigued by the proposal but said his own lab would not make it. He was a scientist and intended to do research, not make a product; in addition, he had no decision-making power in a company the likes of Du Pont. He asked us to write him a letter that he could show to people who controlled budgets.

We did so on September 15, 1982, exactly five years after the trip to Oxford and Japan, when I realized the possibilities IL-2 could open up. It had taken me five years of highly concentrated effort to get this far. But I had hopes that a supply of purified IL-2 would take me much farther much faster.

The letter briefly recounted our animal experiments, pointed out that IL-2 could be an important product, and formally suggested a collaborative project to test IL-2 in people. Robb circulated the letter within the company and visited us. On January 4, 1983, we were informed that Du Pont's director of medical research would let us know the decision.

We did not wait for it. In case the answer was yes, we wanted to be able to move quickly, so we wrote a protocol for clinical trials. These protocols were documents that described the reasons for performing a clinical study and detailed the exact treatments and procedures to be administered to the patients.

By early February, even before Du Pont agreed to cooperate—although it soon did—NCI approved the protocol. In March we began discussions with the Food and Drug Administration about obtaining a designation for IL-2 as an Investigative New Drug, an IND, which is required for most clinical experiments.

Then we told Du Pont we needed 100 milligrams, approximately three and a half ounces, of pure IL-2 for the planned clinical trials. This would require a major commitment of money and resources. The company balked. Arnold Holtzman, Du Pont's director of development, came down to meet with Peter Fischinger, the deputy director of NCI, Mike, and myself and said he wanted NCI to pay for their costs.

I thought this suggestion unreasonable and said so. First, IL-2 was potentially a very important drug. Very important. Second, if IL-2 worked, Du Pont would be marketing it. And the potential market was huge. Third, we would devote laboratory and clinical resources unavailable anywhere else in the world for testing. This would not cost Du Pont a penny.

Holtzman dropped his demand. After we agreed to sign a statement protecting Du Pont from any litigation resulting from treatment, the company began to supply us with IL-2. It was pure but it came in minuscule amounts.

On May 4, 1983, in support of our application for an IND, Du Pont submitted information about its IL-2 preparation to the FDA. Unless the FDA rejects an IND application within thirty days, it is automatically approved. When the thirty days expired we contacted the FDA and they told us to proceed.

On June 20, Rich Robb came to Bethesda and handed us six vials containing 7.5 milligrams, about one-quarter of an ounce, of pure IL-2. He, Mike, and I walked through the lab, then sat down in my office. We were excited. We had never had such a huge amount. It had taken many people working full-time for several months to produce it. I felt almost as if a door had suddenly opened.

We began in vitro testing to make certain it was safe before giving it to patients. Later we received a letter of agreement, signed by Holtzman, which indemnified Du Pont against legal action from patients given their IL-2. But the tone of the letter was enthusiastic. Indeed, there were hints of concern about potential competitors who might try to interest us in using their IL-2. He made clear that he expected us to continue using Du Pont's product as long as it was "suitable," even if other sources became available, "includ[ing] IL-2 made from recombinant sources."

We refused to agree to the stipulation. The word "recombinant" referred to recombinant DNA technology—genetic engineering.

On October 14, 1980, a young biotechnology company named Genentech set a stock market record for the biggest one-day gain of any stock in history: On its first day of public trading its shares went from 35 to 89 in one *hour*. Not long thereafter, another biotechnology company named Cetus Corporation set another stock market record when its initial public offering of stock raised $123 million.

Cetus and Genentech were pioneers in a revolutionary industry built around genetic engineering, and speculators believed they might someday rival IBM, General Motors, and Xerox in size and financial power. Huge amounts of money were at stake. If the promise of genetic engineering is fulfilled, it could revolutionize everything from agriculture to environmental protection to many manufacturing processes.

But the immediate stock market frenzy over the new industry was generated by the promise of interferon, and the race to manufacture it. Like IL-2, interferon is a naturally occurring cytokine, a protein that can inhibit cell growth and stimulate the immune system. Nature produces it in infinitesimal quantities. Recombinant DNA technology could produce it in bulk. At the time the frenzy was over alpha-interferon (there are three kinds of interferon: alpha, beta, and gamma), which was being hailed as a miracle cure, a wonder drug for everything from cancer to the common cold. Unfortunately alpha-interferon turned out not to be a miracle cure, although it has proven to be useful against certain rare cancers.

In the early 1980s, while the race to manufacture interferon was under way, biotechnology companies began looking for other products to make. Interleukin-2 is a lymphokine, a type of cytokine; its name in fact refers to communication between leukocytes, white blood cells. Interleukin-2 was one such possible product.

Cetus, located in Emeryville, California, in the San Francisco Bay area, was not a new company. For some years it had been producing industrial-grade biological products. But its executives understood that the future lay in molecular biology, in manipulating genes to make products. Largely because of the excitement over interferon and other cytokines, they provided capital to a company they named Cetus-Immune in Palo Alto, near the Stanford University campus. This company was started by excellent scientists on the Stanford faculty, including immunologists Hugh McDevitt, Tom Merigan, both on the board of directors of Cetus, and Gary Fathman, who had done his postdoctoral work with my friend Dave Sachs.

I had never heard of Cetus when Fathman called to invite me to give a seminar on my work with IL-2. They had seen my scientific publications and heard other things through the grapevine. I thought that scientists of this caliber might well have ideas that could help me. I might even get them interested in working with IL-2 themselves, which would certainly help me. On July 30, 1982, in the last stages of my series of experiments with partially purified IL-2, I went to Palo Alto.

Cetus-Immune operated out of a small, clean building in a row of what looked like office buildings on a main road. It was unlike any lab I had ever seen. The facility was clean and well equipped but it seemed oddly isolated—one sensed it lacked the creative chaos and collegiality of labs in academic settings. I thought it would be difficult if not impossible to do science this way. But biotech firms were doing science. My listeners seemed to be on a fishing expedition seeking information about IL-2. I was happy to tell them everything I knew, including my latest results and conclusions, which had neither been published nor yet made their way to them through their network of information.

Later I learned that the parent company, Cetus, was then in the process of choosing a new product to make. Along with the Stanford consultants, Cetus scientist David Mark had developed a list of close to sixty possible targets.

The consultants had been excited about IL-2 before my visit. After it, Merigan told me, they got even more excited. In a large meeting the top prospects were written down on a blackboard and discussed. Apparently IL-2 was now the first choice.

On October 20, Cetus invited me to return. IL-2 was more important to me than to them. I knew that recombinant DNA technology could produce it in virtually unlimited amounts. This would end my supply problems. I quickly agreed to return and make a second presentation.

This time the audience was a group of thirty or forty scientists and executives, including several other outside scientists. Afterward I was asked to join the company, become actively involved in their decision-making and planning, and receive stock options. I refused the offer. The Stanford scientists were a little surprised; private universities allow faculty such arrangements. I worked for the government. For me it would be a potential conflict of interest.

It was not the only potential conflict that arose during that visit. After I presented my data, a Cetus scientist began to speak about their efforts to clone the gene for IL-2. The information he was about to present was highly confidential, he said, and had to be kept secret.

I understood their position. They were preparing to commit millions of dollars—ultimately $150 million, a Cetus executive later told me—to develop IL-2 as a commercial product. They did not want their proprietary secrets given to a competitor.

But I was not sympathetic to their position. Secrecy in science has always offended me. The information that Cetus did not want to reveal might help develop effective treatments for cancer.

In that room in California my feelings were particularly strong. I considered it unethical for me to know something that might speed a cure for cancer and not disclose it to anyone who asked. Demands for confidentiality in science remind me of the invention of obstetrical forceps in the seventeenth century by the Chamberlen brothers, who were doctors. They developed a device that could extract an infant from the womb in certain difficult and not uncommon childbirths; before their invention both the mother and child died. But rather than sharing their knowledge freely, they kept it a close secret, selling it to a select few other doctors. All over Europe women and children died while the Chamberlens became rich. Finally a doctor bought the secret and published it. The Chamberlens have been condemned in medicine ever since.

I raised my hand self-consciously—self-conscious only because I did not want to appear self-righteous. I stated that I could not agree to keep anything confidential.

An awkward silence filled the room. Finally a Cetus scientist warned that if I couldn't keep the information confidential, they couldn't tell it to me. I repeated that I could not promise to keep anything secret.

An executive asked me to leave the room. I sat in a scientist's office during the presentation, read scientific papers, and thought about the situation. The emergence of the biotechnology industry was constantly creating conflicts like this between the traditional free exchange of scientific information and the commercial exploitation of that information. At that time, people in other labs began refusing to send me reagents unless I signed a confidentiality statement, which I have never agreed to do. DeWitt Stetten Jr., one of NIH's most respected scientists, had recently written an editorial in *Nature* entitled "The DNA Disease." He pointed out in detail the deleterious impact on communication in science caused by the emergence of the biotechnology industry and took it a step further: "Concurrently a change was noted in the dissertation problems assigned to graduate students. Whereas formerly they always contained an element of new knowledge, now the stress is on a new product, and preferably a marketable one."

Science has always been part of the world and never wholly innocent. But it had been a special part of the world. It was losing some of its specialness.

As I thought about this I also thought how stupid it was for me to be sitting outside. I could help them in that room. While others had studied the basic science of IL-2 more than I had, no one else in the world had as much practical experience with it. It drove home to me that Cetus was in this to make money. And it taught me never to be naive in my dealings with a biotech company.

At the same time, Cetus was pouring money into the project. We were serving each other's purposes. It was a risk for them and a very large risk. They had no way to know if IL-2 would ever work. Neither did I.

But if the risk was large, so could be the return. The race to manufacture IL-2 was on. The competitors included Hoffman-La Roche, Amgen, Genentech, Du Pont, and Cetus. The winner was hoping for hundreds of millions of dollars in profits.

Cetus was determined to win that race. And winning required the mastery of recombinant DNA technology and of molecular biology, the foundations upon which the entire biotechnology industry was being constructed—and which penetrated to the nature of life itself.

Cetus occupied an old, remodeled Shell Oil engineering facility built in the 1930s, with thick concrete walls, a linoleum floor, and a suspended ceiling of acoustic tiles. The lobby was dominated by a huge mural of a whale—the symbol of Cetus—jumping over the Golden Gate Bridge. Another mural showed a Berkeley scene with people surprised by the sudden suspension of gravity. As then Cetus scientist Ed Bradley, who came from the East Coast and later returned there, observed, "It was a cross between Escher and Norman Rockwell. Very California. Very Berkeley."

But from what I understand there was nothing laid-back about the intensity with which Cetus pursued IL-2. As the project advanced, leadership of it rotated, from David Mark, a molecular biologist who ran the genetic engineering aspects, to Kirston Koths, a protein chemist responsible for making a clinically acceptable molecule and scaling up production, to Bradley, who helped run the clinical trials, to business-oriented executives. Attendees to weekly meetings changed too, beginning with only scientists and finally including patent attorneys. The project managers kept everything on the track of what they called "the critical path from clone to clinic."

The first step was to clone the gene for IL-2. A gene is really nothing more than a stretch of information written in a chemical code and contained in the DNA molecule. The information itself dictates the production of one—and only one—protein.

A gene is like software that tells the machinery of the cell what to do. Once the gene is cloned, it can be inserted into bacteria. It would order each bacterium to become a tiny factory churning out the desired protein.

Cetus lost the race to clone the gene for IL-2. A Japanese scientist named Tadatsugu Taniguchi isolated it from the Jurkat cell line in late 1982 and put it into monkey cells; the cells began making low levels of IL-2. He showed the slide of the sequence at a scientific meeting and got a dramatic reaction. Shortly thereafter he published the gene's sequence in *Nature*.

But rather than give up, Cetus accelerated its efforts. David Mark is a very short, very intense man. Although pleasant, with him everything is to the point. He and other company scientists quickly got the gene from Jurkat IL-2 and also from normal human lymphocytes. The two genes made identical proteins.

Mark then inserted the gene into bacteria. A common bacteria called *E. coli* was used. The bacterial cell was transformed. As a result, 5 to 10 percent of all the protein produced by these transformed *E. coli* was IL-2.

But no one knew whether the engineered protein would perform the same way as the natural one. Natural IL-2 was bound to many sugar molecules. Recombinant IL-2 made by bacteria was not bound to sugars. Also, Cetus scientists had changed one amino acid in the recombinant IL-2 to make it more stable.

Kirston Koths at Cetus took charge of demonstrating that the recombinant molecule functioned properly and designing a way to produce it in commercial quantities. Koths superficially seems the opposite of Mark. Tall, thin, with long hair sometimes tied in a ponytail and a somewhat disheveled throwback-to-the-sixties appearance, there is a sense about him that he marches to his own drummer. But if his style is laid-back, he is an excellent scientist, very straightforward and, like Mark, to the point. Belying his appearance is a quotation on his wall: "Good. Fast. Cheap. Pick two."

Koths had three simple, but not easy, goals: to make the purest recombinant protein possible that could be scaled up to commercial production; to have it function as much like the natural protein as possible; and to do this fast.

In his lab he received ten liters of concentrated bacteria, which resembled frozen butterscotch pudding wrapped in Saran Wrap. Six weeks later, after roaring through and solving a dozen complications with what he called his "polishing steps," he had concentrated the IL-2 and partially purified it.

By May 1983, his chief concern was scaling up the effort. He was making recombinant IL-2 in batches 100,000 times the amounts of natural IL-2 we were making. And he had to make it in still larger quantities.

In mid-June, Cetus held an annual retreat for all its scientists. The company asked me to give a lecture on June 12 about my own latest experiments with IL-2. I went reluctantly and planned to leave immediately after my presentation to catch the red-eye flight back to Washington. The retreat astounded me.

It was held at a hotel on the beach south of San Francisco, and more than 100 Cetus scientists and many outsiders attended. The surroundings seemed, to me at least, sumptuous. Cetus was obviously pouring money into this event and, even more, into its IL-2 effort. Looking around, for the first time I fully comprehended the enormity of the company's commitment to IL-2. I was later told that the Cetus investment was then approaching $50 million—and rising.

This flat-out commitment, decided upon by Robert Fildes, its chief executive officer, was an enormous gamble for Cetus and it registered on me. Cetus scientists knew less than I did about IL-2's potential practical applications, and I still knew almost nothing. At this point I did not even know if LAK cells could cure metastases. I was gambling my own professional life on IL-2. They were gambling the company.

I gave my talk in the afternoon and presented all my best data and dreams for the future. My impression was that I had stunned most of the scientists in the audience, and that Cetus had actually invited me to talk to use me to motivate their people. My results may have made them feel that they were attacking cancer, not simply putting out a product. They were already working hard. I gave them a reason to work harder.

Francis Crick, one of the great scientific minds of the century and a discoverer of the structure of DNA, was in the audience. I had never met him but we talked briefly after my presentation. Then I walked out, anxious to get to the airport and home.

Kirston Koths was walking with me. It was dusk. Earlier in the day I had asked about the chances of getting some of the recombinant IL-2. I had been put off. Later I learned that my request had forced a decision in the company as to whether to collaborate with me or not, and that this was an extremely controversial point within Cetus and remained so for some years. Some in the company were concerned that, as I had demonstrated when I objected to their request for confidentiality, they would have no control—and they would not have any—over how I used their IL-2 if they gave it to me. To them, recombinant IL-2 was like a baby. They feared that some of my experiments might reflect badly on their product. They also feared that my needs would devour nearly all the IL-2 they produced, inevitably if inadvertently cutting out other researchers. They would then have to live or die on the basis of my work. This possible dependence on me made them uncomfortable.

Others wanted to collaborate. They argued that their goal was a clinical trial—that was the whole point of their "critical path" management approach—and that no investigator in the world had the commitment I had to using immune approaches to treat cancer, while no institution in the world could match the clinical resources of NCI. Jeff Price, the president, made the decision.

At the time I knew nothing of this internal Cetus debate. Now, outside the hotel, as I was about to step into a car to the airport, I learned the outcome. I told Koths I wanted some IL-2.

He smiled. "Okay, I have some for you."

He reached into his pocket and pulled out a screw-top test tube with scribblings on it containing a clear liquid. He was apologetic, warning me it was a fraction just coming off a column, filled with impurities. "Frankly, this is crap," he said. "We can do better."

"Don't worry," I assured him. "As soon as you have better stuff, send it. Meanwhile let's see how good this is."

He briefly detailed its impurities to give me an idea of what to expect. Then he handed me the test tube. I put it in the breast pocket of my suit jacket, thinking this was very strange.

It was to me a huge amount, more than I had ever had at one time, what seemed to me the world's supply of IL-2—and I was storing it in my jacket pocket. I tried to hide my excitement. Then Koths said he had much more back in the lab. I grew more excited.

Yet I also knew that the recombinant product was not exactly the same as natural IL-2. I had no idea whether it would work. I had no idea whether it would grow T cells, or make LAK cells, or by itself affect cancers.

But I was going to find out, and quickly.

Kirston gave me the vial on June 12, and I flew back across the country through the night. On June 14, I started two experiments simultaneously, and on June 15, a third.

The first experiment would assess the ability of recombinant IL-2, rIL-2, to make T cells grow. The second measured its effects on in vitro sensitization of T cells against foreign cells. The third tested its ability to make LAK cells.

In each of these experiments we used several different titers, or concentrations, of the protein. Within a few days we had the results. When we grew cells in the lab, we very rarely used purified IL-2. It was too precious to waste on this task. Generally we used the lectin-free IL-2 supe at dilutions of 1:2 or 1:4. *The recombinant IL-2 could grow cells at dilutions of 1:400,000.*

The in vitro sensitization experiment—repeating what we had done in the first *if*—yielded encouraging results, but nothing dramatic. But on June 20 we got the LAK results. Natural lectin-free IL-2 generally could not make good LAK cells at dilutions greater than 1:2. *rIL-2 made good LAK cells at dilutions of 1:2,500.*

I started more experiments but quickly ran out of rIL-2, called Koths on June 23, told him the results, and asked for more. I had it the next day by overnight air express. Soon we were performing in vivo experiments in mice. The recombinant IL-2's half-life was 2.8 minutes, which was comparable to that of natural IL-2.

In every experiment, the recombinant IL-2 behaved exactly like natural lectin-free IL-2—except that the recombinant material was immensely more potent because it was immensely purer.

If I could get continued access to this recombinant material, supplies of IL-2 would never be a problem again.

Earlier I had felt as if there was a powerful machine at my disposal, that its engine was ready to roar, but that I could not find the key to it—and that the key lay hidden somewhere in the lab. I had wondered if IL-2 was that key.

Now I would find out. Now I might also find out whether my hypothesis—that we could take immune system cells out of the body, grow them, and use them to cure a cancer—was true.

My impatience for the answer became difficult to control. Everything was moving quickly now. Each day we seemed to learn something new. As I parked the car in the NIH garage each morning, I would head for the stairs—the elevator took too long—and discover that within a few steps I was almost running, that I was taking the stairs two and three at a time, that I was arriving at my lab already out of breath, already impatient to begin.

CHAPTER THIRTEEN

T he lab became a beehive. It hummed and buzzed. One could almost *hear* the intensity. As we defined the capabilities and characteristics of recombinant IL-2 from Cetus, the pace of our footsteps quickened, our movements became more jerky, as if everything took too long and we could somehow hasten the pace of the world if we ourselves moved faster.

Yet I felt increasingly buffeted. As I sat at my desk, outside my office to the right, in the lab, all was hope and eagerness. But to the left, down the hall in the hospital ward, our patients continued to die. I could not allow my enthusiasm for the one or my discouragement over the other to affect me or those around me. The only way to maintain an evenness of temperament was to focus more intently on my work. I did.

I ended the clinical protocol giving patients lectin-activated killer cells. We had treated twenty-one people. Not one had shown any benefit from the treatment. We had only raised their hopes, and our own, and then watched them die. We had, however, learned much about repeated phereses, culturing large numbers of cells, and giving these cells to patients.

Mike Lotze and I got Du Pont's highly purified, natural IL-2 on June 20, 1983, a week after Kirston Koths handed me the first raw Cetus recombinant material. While I began to test this recombinant IL-2 in the laboratory, we also prepared to give the natural IL-2—the only material the FDA had approved for human trials—to the first patient.

I had first met Sheila Hopeland seven years earlier, when she was sixty-two years old. There were two unusual things about her. Though a small, even frail, woman and very quiet, she seemed so gentle that paradoxically she had a powerful presence. One felt good being near her. She also had quite beautiful shoulder-length brown hair, longer than I have ever seen in a woman her age; it made her seem younger than her years.

She initially came to us during one of our early randomized protocols for patients with primary melanomas. She had randomized to the standard treatment; we performed a wide excision of her tumor and removed lymph nodes from her groin, which were negative. On the basis of this and the nature of her tumor, she had a 60 percent chance of being cured.

Unfortunately, within a year new lesions appeared in her leg. We removed them but they kept recurring. She received chemotherapy at the University of Maryland. It failed. She received more chemotherapy. The cancer grew. She received radiation therapy. The disease spread.

By now Mrs. Hopeland had extensive disease. She had failed repeated surgery, chemotherapy, and radiation. There was nothing left to do.

I spoke to her. She was struggling to appear vigorous. Her struggle made her seem both more frail and more gentle. We offered her the IL-2. Quietly she agreed to become our first patient to receive it.

On July 20, 1983, we placed her in the Intensive Care Unit and prepared the first dose. We had no way of knowing how best to give it, and the protocol allowed us to infuse it continuously, dripping it gradually into a vein over a twenty-four-hour period once a week, or to give a bolus injection, intravenously, over a thirty-minute period once a week. In both cases we could slowly escalate the dosage.

Two Australian investigators had previously given two patients minute amounts of IL-2. We also began Mrs. Hopeland with a minuscule dose by bolus injection—14 micrograms, or 14 millionths of a gram. In the experiments in which we had seen IL-2's anticancer activity, mice had received doses several thousand times greater in proportion to their weight.

Although neither Mike Lotze nor I expected any side effects, we hovered about her in the ICU, along with Claudia Seipp, my chief research nurse, whom I had hired soon after coming to NIH. There were in fact no side effects.

She received four doses, one a week. There were no effects of any kind. Mrs. Hopeland died of her disease a short time later.

On July 26, we started our second patient on IL-2. On August 2, a twenty-two-year-old boy named Raul Fernandez began treatment. It was my forty-third birthday.

That night Alice had a small party for me. I tried to separate my two lives and smiled my way through the party and the good wishes of a few friends. But my mind was on Mr. Fernandez and the party was flat. My friends left early. At 10:00 I returned to the hospital. Working made me feel better.

I call Mr. Fernandez a boy because I think of him as one. He had lived through more than most of us see in a long lifetime, and he seemed an odd combination of child and man, part Oliver Twist and part Fagan. He was Puerto Rican, from New York City, and one of twelve children. From the age of one and a half he had lived in foster homes. His mother visited him regularly until he was nine, when she was murdered by his father, whom he neither knew nor had any desire to know. He was not in contact with a single relative on either side of his family. Our social worker observed, "He is a rough and streetwise kid."

On the surface he seemed unreliable. When he was admitted to the hospital shortly before treatment, we sent him downstairs to get X rays for preliminary studies; he failed to show up there and did not return that day. Yet he did not seem a bad kid. He had had numerous homosexual contacts but said that his promiscuity was not a preference but a means of survival. Maybe he considered the X rays irrelevant, for our convenience and not his, saw us as using him, and he was tired of being used. If rough and streetwise, he did not live either off or in the streets and had made a living in New York as a late-night disc jockey at a small radio station. A year before he came to us, he had moved to Virginia. There he had found what he called the first loving relationship of his life with a man thirty-five years older than he.

A local doctor had diagnosed Kaposi's sarcoma, a normally rare cancer associated with the new disease AIDS, and referred him to NIH. Mr. Fernandez had AIDS. Little was known in 1983 about the disease except that it affected the immune system, and five of the first ten patients to receive IL-2 were AIDS patients with Kaposi's sarcoma. He told us he had always had to struggle for survival and would struggle through this. "I'm going to get my life together," he added.

I vividly recall him saying that. I believed he meant that he knew he was dying.

He too received a trivial dose of IL-2, one one-hundredth what mice had received. It had no effect on his cancer or his AIDS.

By the fifth patient, we had raised the dose to 1,000 micrograms, or one milligram. We had only 7.5 milligrams and were administering almost one-seventh our entire supply in one dose. It was still not enough to see any antitumor effects, although it did cause some immunologic changes.

We desperately needed more IL-2.

Not everyone agreed. A prominent member of the National Academy of Sciences attacked us for using purified IL-2 in clinical trials. He told Mike Lotze that IL-2 should be studied only in the lab until better understood. "How can you be throwing away this IL-2 on patients?" he demanded. "It's so precious."

It *was* precious, terribly precious. After we ran out of the first batch, Du Pont sent another 17 milligrams on December 20, 1983—a Christmas present, Rich Robb said—and in February 1984, another 10 milligrams. That was all we would get. The largest single dose we gave anyone was 2 milligrams by bolus injection. We saw fever and chills, and for the first time some liver abnormalities, which quickly returned to normal.

We needed more IL-2.

.   .   .

As these trials proceeded, I was pushing our work in the laboratory forward. In 1983 Maury Rosenstein left and I missed him. He had arrived interested in science but decided that he wanted to apply his knowledge clinically and go to medical school. I encouraged him. He went to Bowman-Grey Medical School in Winston-Salem, North Carolina, and often called me on Saturday afternoons, when he knew I would be relatively alone. We would talk about the latest experiments and our future plans. Later he returned to the lab for one summer and did some excellent work. He is now on the faculty of radiation therapy of the University of Pittsburgh.

I was very sorry to see Maury leave. I was very pleased when Jim Mulé arrived from the Fred Hutchinson Cancer Center in Seattle to replace him.

From Jim's first letter to me inquiring about a position, I found the cohesiveness of his thoughts impressive. His language was informal but his words fitted snugly together; they suggested both a depth of understanding and an ability to see forests. Even before joining our lab—at a time when tumor immunology was still outside the mainstream—he knew not only what he wanted to pursue, but how it fitted into my own plans.

There was nothing flashy about him; instead, he seemed low-key, mature, and stable. Thin but not intense, he smiled frequently and seemed more likely to shrug his shoulders over a disagreement than get into an argument. He made a point of identifying himself as Sicilian, had a strong sense of family and place, and came from a blue-collar background in New Jersey. Most people in the lab went to elite universities and as children had planned careers in science or medicine; Jim went to Jersey City State College, played in a rock band, and expected to teach high school biology. Fortunately one of his professors urged him to go to graduate school.

Jim's maturity helped stabilize the lab and served as a soothing presence for everyone. Yet if much about him seemed laid-back and frictionless, Jim was easy to underestimate. He was also not to be underestimated. His focus and sense of purpose could burn through obstacles. He reminded me of a basketball player who so fits into the flow of a game that one barely notices his presence; then, seeing that he scored thirty-two points, one realizes that this player had, through passes and intelligence rather than dunks, controlled the flow of the game and made those around him more productive. Jim's own work was outstanding, and he would later become the only Ph.D. ever to be granted tenure in the Surgery Branch.

Yet his experience here did not start well. I wanted him to extend Amitabha Mazumder's work—in which LAK cells alone, without any IL-2, had cured mice of the B16 melanoma—by seeing if the LAK cells worked against larger tumor burdens, if adding chemotherapeutic agents made treatment more effective, and if other adjustments improved results. He began by trying to replicate Amitabha's findings. He could not.

He was a young investigator, brand-new to the lab and in his first real job. His failures made him doubt his own abilities. I recall one Sunday each of us sitting in our chairs, recording results from our different experiments. He could tell just from glancing at the vials that the LAK cells had failed again to cure the melanoma in the animals. He swore in frustration.

I was frustrated, too. Those frustrations would soon dissipate.

Through the summer and fall of 1983, as the clinical trials with natural IL-2 were ongoing without effect, as Jim Mulé was experiencing failures, I experimented with the Cetus material. I would exhaust the supply rapidly, call Kirston Koths, and he would ship his latest batch by overnight express. For weeks we went on like this, hand to mouth. Each shipment varied in potency and we had to establish its titer ourselves, but each shipment continued to behave exactly as did Du Pont's purified natural IL-2—except that the recombinant material was available in immensely larger amounts than the natural product.

Still, my first experimental therapies in mice in August and early September showed mixed results at best. Sue Schwarz and I were injecting animals with B16 melanoma cells, then treating them with rIL-2. We were getting some antitumor effects but in a scattered pattern that was not statistically significant. Chance alone could have accounted for the positive results.

I thought the problem might be the B16 melanoma model. I had originally asked Amitabha to use this tumor because we were casting about for any model that would yield useful information. I had never been comfortable using the B16 tumor because it had existed in culture for so many years, and I was certain it had developed unnatural properties that affected experimental results. I decided to abandon my work with it. I did have Jim Mulé continue his work with B16, only because Amitabha had used it and Jim was trying to repeat and extend Amitabha's results.

For my own experiments, I jumped ahead to another tumor model, the MCA-100 sarcoma series. I believed that of all laboratory cancers, this model most closely represented the kind of disease that occurred naturally in people, and we took care to avoid letting these cancer cells mutate and develop unnatural properties. The MCA-100 tumors were also particularly vicious and aggressive cancers; they offered a hard test for any potential therapy.

On September 9, I set up an experiment with Paul Spiess involving four different MCA-100 tumor lines and treated the mice with rIL-2 in a 1:7,000 dilution, LAK cells, and the chemotherapeutic agent cyclophosphamide. Paul injected tumor cells subcutaneously, under the skin, where they grew. Later we saw some very slight decreases in tumors in some IL-2-treated animals. These decreases were not statistically significant and barely suggested an antitumor effect.

But that same day Sue and I started another experiment with just one sarcoma cell line, MCA-105. It was to be an experiment that changed the course of our work.

Instead of injecting tumor cells under the skin, as in Paul's experiment, I injected fresh MCA-105 tumor cells intravenously. These cancer cells circulated in the bloodstream. The first capillary bed, the first small blood vessel, these cells encountered was in the lung, and the cells lodged there. We waited three days for tumors to establish themselves.

Then we broke the animals into five groups. One control group received nothing. Another control group received 80 million fresh lymphocytes. And three groups received treatments we believed might have some effect: One group received a single injection of 80 million LAK cells; one group received recombinant IL-2 alone, injected intraperitoneally—into the belly, where it was slowly absorbed by the body—three times a day for three days; and one group received both 80 million LAK cells *and* the IL-2 injections.

Sue ear-tagged all the animals with a metal clip and wrote down the number of the mouse and the treatment it received. This was the code, which she then placed in an envelope and sealed. In my lab the person performing the experiment cannot keep the envelope containing the code—I want no one tempted to glance at the code, which could create unconscious bias—so she gave it to Jim Mulé to hold.

On September 23, fourteen days after first injecting the tumor cells, Sue sacrificed the animals. She then opened the chest and, using a technique developed by Hilda Wexler at NIH several years earlier, she injected India ink into the trachea. This turns the lungs black, but the tumors do not absorb the ink. After bleaching, the tumors show up white against the black background of the lung. Sue extracted the lungs, counted the number of metastases on each lung, and wrote the number down next to the ear-tag number for each mouse.

This was tedious and took time. I asked Sue to break the code with Jim Mulé and come into my office as soon as she had tabulated the results.

Sue's work area is immediately outside my door, literally a few steps from my desk. My door was open. She walked in holding a piece of paper, looking down at it as she spoke. "I think it might have had an effect," she said, "but I'm not sure."

She handed me the sheet of paper. I read the results, then stood up. Something in the pattern of the numbers told me that these results were no coincidence, that they were unlike anything we had ever seen. Thunderbolt moments do not happen often in research—sometimes they come years apart and many scientists never experience even one—but when they occur they make any amount of previous failure seem trivial. And one knows such a moment instantly.

The animals that had received no treatment had an average of 42 metastases.

Those that had received fresh lymphocytes had an average of 63 mets.

LAK cells alone, 38 mets.

IL-2 alone, 40 mets.

LAK and IL-2 in combination, 22 mets.

Perhaps more important was the fact that there was no overlap. None at all. The lowest number of mets in any untreated animal was 35. The highest number of mets in any animal treated with both LAK cells and IL-2 was 32. And one of the animals treated with LAK and IL-2 had no mets at all. Its cancer was gone.

This was a thunderbolt moment. My first reaction was an intellectual one as I recognized the meaning of the results. Then that meaning deepened, flowed through me, became visceral.

The relatively small decrease in tumors in treated compared with untreated mice might not have impressed others in the lab. Yet my experience of having stared in disappointment at results from all my previous failed experiments allowed me to recognize immediately that this result was different. The pattern of the LAK and IL-2 group was special. I felt certain that the result was statistically significant.

"This looks real," I said.

It was all that needed to be said.

This looks real. The hypothesis I had formulated years earlier predicted this result. And here it was. The very first time we used LAK cells and IL-2 together to treat our most vicious sarcomas, it worked. We were seeing results in the very first experiment, long before we had optimized our technique of performing it.

I was excited but did not want to act excited. I feared the result might not repeat. Yet I was confident it would. My hesitancy was habit. I am the most skeptical person in our lab. The fellows come in excited and often all I say is, "Do it again." But I believed this result. *This is real,* I said to myself. *This is real. We will see this result again.*

Within minutes after Sue came into my office and handed me her tabulations, we set up a repeat of the experiment.

Every night at dinner my daughters, Alice, and I go around the table and explain what happened to each of us that day. Usually I go last. That night I took my turn first. My daughters were then too young to understand; counting the number of lung metastases in mice did not excite them. But they understood that I was excited. And Alice understood all that this meant.

That first experiment proved to have a P value of .02, which meant that there was only a 2 percent likelihood that chance accounted for the results. A 98 percent likelihood existed that the treatment had worked. Normally, any P value less than .05 is considered statistically significant.

On October 14, 1983, we surpassed the first result by an enormous margin. I used three different kinds of IL-2—our lectin-free IL-2 supe produced our old way, IL-2 from the high-producing EL-4 mouse cell line, and the recombinant material—and varied the dilutions so they were of equal potency. I wanted this experiment to be unquestioned and so Sue and I, as a check on each other, each counted mets independently. Although our counts did not agree exactly—each of us had to judge, for example, whether an irregular greyish spot was two separate small tumors or a single larger one—our overall results did.

The control animals had an average of forty-eight mets each by my count, forty-seven by Sue's.

The animals treated with LAK cells and IL-2—no matter what the source of the IL-2—averaged less than one tumor each. More than half of the treated mice, including five of the six animals given recombinant IL-2 along with LAK, had no tumors at all.

It appeared that their cancers had been cured.

We had answered the fourth *if* definitively. We had taken

immune system cells from a tumor-bearing animal—an animal with cancer—changed them in culture, and then returned the cells to the animal, where they attacked, and destroyed, the cancer.

The one remaining *if*, the fifth one, required doing the same thing in man.

While Sue performed experiments with the LAK cells plus IL-2, Paul and I were exploring the potency of rIL-2 alone. On November 7, we set up a large experiment with numerous controls and several different dosages of rIL-2, without LAK cells. In animals receiving the largest dosage—an amount vastly greater than the IL-2 we were giving to our patients in the clinical trials—well-established subcutaneous tumors stopped growing.

Every good scientist is his or her own most brutal critic, and I recognized that there were some unlikely but theoretically possible explanations for these results. We did more experiments and ruled out these theoretical explanations. Only one explanation remained: Recombinant IL-2 in very large doses impacted on cancer.

Following this work, the lab erupted in an enormous flurry of activity, all of it revolving around rIL-2. Much later Paul did a half-serious computation and estimated that over the next year the drops of recombinant IL-2 left in the bottom of test tubes that we threw out were equivalent to the amount of natural IL-2 we could have gotten from killing 900 million mice.

We were pouring rIL-2 into animals, learning about it, exploring its limits. Later Jim Mulé, commenting on the extraordinary number of papers that people in the lab were publishing in major journals, said, "It was like being on the 1961 Yankees."

Through this period, while those working solely in the lab were rife with excitement and flooded with supplies of rIL-2, Mike Lotze was running the clinical trials with Du Pont's purified natural IL-2. The company had promised to supply us with 100 milligrams of pure IL-2, but they encountered serious production problems with contamination and purification. Du Pont took more than a year to make 34.5 milligrams, which was all they could ever deliver to us.

Du Pont's natural IL-2 and the Cetus recombinant material were comparable in concentration and potency. They had comparable effects on cells and in patients. The only difference was, Mike calculated, that it had taken thirty people working full-time for approximately one year to refine those 34.5 milligrams from 10,000 liters of supernatant.

One liter of easy-to-grow bacteria could produce 100 milligrams of recombinant IL-2 in days.

Until the emergence of recombinant DNA technology, few investigators in biology had interacted directly with industry. That had changed. My experience with Cetus showed me both positive and negative outgrowths of this new interaction. If the increased secrecy in science disturbed me, the efforts of Cetus scientists were now complementing my own. It would have been impossible for me to produce large quantities of recombinant IL-2 in my lab without stopping all other work and devoting all my resources to it. But Cetus had produced it, and the company had taken a large risk in doing so. Cetus and other biotechnology companies were working with other investigators in other labs as well. Symbiotic relationships were being created.

The race was over. Cetus had won it. And we too had won.

The new biotechnology industry had also shown its power, and the power of recombinant DNA technology. Cetus had made a product in quantities impossible for Du Pont, one of the world's largest chemical companies, to duplicate by traditional production methods. And recombinant IL-2 only hinted at the potential of this new industry.

In early March 1984, we used the last of our Du Pont supply. We treated a total of sixteen patients with it. I remember each one. A metallurgist from Ohio with five children from two to twenty-two. A twenty-five-year-old music student from Florida. A sixty-two-year-old laundry worker from Rhode Island. No patient's cancer responded to treatment. All soon died of their disease.

We had long before begun the process of seeking FDA approval to use the recombinant material in clinical trials, and we received approval on January 17, 1984, only seven months after Kirston Koths gave me the first test tube of rIL-2, contaminated with endotoxins and other impurities. No one had any idea then if it would work at all, much less how well. Now we were preparing to put it into people.

The Cetus scientists were exuberant and soon sent us a large batch of rIL-2 to give patients. Cetus was clearly gearing up for massive production. That first test tube had been small, clear, and ordinary-looking, with scratchings on the outside in Kirston's handwriting. The first shipments had varied widely in potency. This shipment came in powdered form in neat vials of FDA-approved packaging, with a consistent potency. We promptly began a series of tests on the batch we would use clinically to guarantee it was active and contained no contaminants.

Meanwhile we evaluated what we had learned from the first sixteen patients who had received the natural IL-2. We had learned much.

We discovered that the half-life of IL-2 in people was five to seven minutes, barely longer than in mice, which confirmed that we would need enormous quantities for an effective therapy. And although we had not been able to give high enough doses to see significant toxicities, we had observed changes in hormone levels, minor fluid loss and weight gain, and abnormal liver function. These side effects warned us of potential future complications. And we learned several things that seemed strange. We were particularly interested in one unanticipated finding.

We had expected an increase in the number of lymphocytes after IL-2 was administered. Instead, within minutes of administration, lymphocytes and all LAK precursors disappeared from the blood.

The lymphocytes could not be dying off that quickly. They had to be leaving the bloodstream. This was very interesting. To attack a tumor, lymphocytes would have to leave the bloodstream. The lymphocytes later reappeared in the blood in larger numbers as treatment continued—a rebound effect.

Because we were studying people, we could not learn where the lymphocytes had gone. We could not, for example, take a sample of tissue from a patient just to learn if it was infiltrated by lymphocytes. Even if a patient is willing, medical ethics do not allow a doctor to do anything harmful just because the doctor wants to know something. Only in animals can we answer such questions. All we could study was the patients' blood. That is one reason experimental animals are so important; in animals we can answer questions impossible to answer in man.

We published paper after paper on clinical science—on the physiology of patients after the administration of cytokines. It was extraordinarily productive.

Less productive was my first embroilment in bureaucratic politics, and it later became apparent that more would be at stake than turf. We had treated patients with Du Pont's natural IL-2 after FDA approval, and the FDA had now approved treatment with recombinant IL-2.

Treatment with killer cells was a separate issue. Killer cells were not a drug. They were produced in my lab using lectin-free IL-2 supe. We had gotten approval from an NIH review committee for this treatment without consulting the FDA, which had no authority over it.

Now the FDA insisted on approving treatment with LAK cells generated by rIL-2 because the rIL-2 came from California. The FDA has jurisdiction over material shipped over a state line, and it wanted to establish its authority. My inclination was to resist, but Vincent DeVita, director of NCI and a close friend, decided that since we were a government agency we should submit. Vince has never been afraid to fight but in this case declined because he did not want to set a precedent that private industry would note. I respected his judgment and agreed.

On March 21, 1984, the FDA approved our giving LAK cells generated with rIL-2 to patients.

But the FDA would not allow us to give LAK cells in combination with rIL-2.

We could treat patients with either rIL-2 or LAK cells, but not both simultaneously. We had to show that each alone was safe before the FDA would approve the combination. Yet we achieved our best results in animal models giving both simultaneously. For the moment, in my eagerness to begin, I put that frustration aside.

We finished our lab testing of the first batch of Cetus material for contaminants. There were no problems. We finally had an unlimited supply of IL-2. We were now ready to administer it to patients.

CHAPTER FOURTEEN

On the NIH campus, buildings are known by numbers, not names. Building 10 is the Clinical Center, and in it are both the hospital and my labs. Directly across the street from it is an NIH apartment complex reserved for clinicians who must respond instantly to patient emergencies. When Jim Mulé arrived, I arranged for him to rent there because he routinely had to inject mice in the middle of the night. But he was not the only person in the lab who came in at odd hours. No investigator works a formal shift, and some have always preferred working at midnight, or at 2:00 A.M., or at 4:00 A.M. The silence then is exhilarating; one can concentrate with an intensity impossible during the day. They worked in bursts of thirty-six hours at a stretch, sometimes longer, before going home to sleep. As the people in the lab changed, as different individuals responded to the pull of the night, the membership of this night crew has changed, but it has always existed.

Jim belonged to this night crew when he arrived. He and Steve Ettinghausen, then a surgical fellow, used to go out together on weekends. Jim often joked about being in a Georgetown bar, having a conversation with several young women, when Steve would say, "We've got to take off. We have dates with thirty ladies in fur coats."

Invariably the women, now curious, were invited to come along, and they soon found themselves in the mouse room in the middle of the night. This room can seem a strange and confining place; steel racks, not unlike those in college cafeterias on which students leave trays, fill the room, allowing only enough space for a narrow walkway and the workbench. Each level of each rack is filled with plastic metal-framed cages, usually six mice to a cage, and the room smells of animals. The women would watch while Steve and Jim pulled out cage after cage of mice, lifted one at a time by its tail, held it rigidly, injected it, and returned it—all so quickly that the mouse could not climb its tail and bite. Jim once commented a little sadly, "Steve always seemed to have high hopes but I never saw one of the women come back."

Jim needed such relief. Months after coming to the lab, he was still trying and still failing to replicate Amitabha Mazumder's work curing mice of B16 melanoma with LAK cells alone.

I did not believe the failures were his fault. Nor did I think they reflected on Amitabha, who had repeated the experiment several times under blinded conditions. Jim's inability to reproduce it was one of those strange things that occur in a lab when one is dealing with questions as complex and poorly understood as the growth of a tumor in a living animal. Factors over which one has little control can change and have unexpected, imponderable effects—changes as varied as contamination of the transplanted tumor, or the temperature in the animal room, or a supplier altering its preparation of a reagent.

It seemed a waste of Jim's energy and my resources to have him devote more time to working on the B16 model. I asked him if he wanted to abandon B16 and take over the series of experiments Sue and I had started, and in which we had gotten startling results by using LAK cells in conjunction with rIL-2 against the MCA-100 sarcomas.

He was ecstatic at the prospect.

We never did find out why LAK cells stopped curing the B16 cancers. But he dove into his new work almost vengefully, taking out his frustrations from all the failures in the other experimental system.

Jim quickly familiarized himself with the model by replicating what Sue and I had done, and then quickly moved past it. His successes were dramatic—so dramatic that our code-breaking ceremonies ended. As almost every experiment worked as predicted and the suspense dissipated, the ceremonies became anti-climactic. But the findings were not anticlimactic.

The resulting paper written by Jim, along with Suyu Shu, a research fellow in the lab, Sue and myself, reported on the effect of LAK cells and IL-2 on cancers. It was a solid and comprehensive paper that characterized the phenomenon fully and described the role of recombinant IL-2 in detail as well. We had demonstrated that recombinant IL-2 and LAK cells eliminated cancer in animals.

Specialization in science has created communication problems. Often findings relevant to several fields get lost because they are published in a specialized journal read only by scientists working in only one area. I believed this paper was important not only for immunologists to read, but also for scientists in other areas. I wanted the broadest possible audience. If the paper generated the same excitement in other investigators that I felt, then others might begin working in related areas and speed progress significantly. The two most widely read scientific journals in the world are *Science*, published by the American Association for the Advancement of Science, and the British journal *Nature*. For Jim, a young investigator doing his first major work, publication in either journal would mark a major milestone.

For no reason that I can recall, I chose to submit our paper to *Nature* in early 1984. An editor rejected it with a standard form letter saying it did "not have sufficient general interest to warrant publication in *Nature*" and suggested sending it to a specialty journal.

Jim was disturbed and worried that the work might not be as important as we thought. I was disturbed, too, but for another reason. Their comment made little sense to me and reflected a bias against clinical, as opposed to basic, science. I told Jim, "I guess they don't consider treating cancer of general interest."

On March 4, before we treated the first patient with recombinant IL-2, we submitted the paper to *Science*. Jim was antsy. Six weeks later he asked me about it and I suggested he call the journal to find out what their decision was. A few minutes later

Jim walked in beaming and told me *Science* had accepted the paper. I jumped up and shook his hand.

Even as this paper was being accepted, our knowledge of LAK cells and IL-2, both in combination and apart, was exploding. Jim performed elegant experiments on the mechanism of action of the LAK cells. Steve Ettinghausen showed that LAK cells grew in mice—inside the animals—when IL-2 was given. Rene Lafreniere, a Canadian, showed that LAK cells and IL-2 worked in a different model system against liver metastases, which strongly implied the result would hold true in other situations as well. Eitan Shiloni, an Israeli, reproduced many of these results using LAK cells in different mouse strains, further suggesting that our results might represent a general principle. Jim Yang, a surgical fellow, identified the LAK subpopulations that actually did the killing. Moshe Papa, another Israeli, showed that IL-2 plus chemotherapy yielded better results than either did alone. And John Vetto demonstrated that steroids inhibited the activity of IL-2.

We published thirty-two papers that year, and forty-four the next—almost one a week. Each paper reflected our deepening understanding of both the science involved and the likely effects on patients.

And the last sentence of our paper in *Science* read, "Clinical trials of the infusion of LAK cells generated with rIL-2 as well as Phase I trials of the infusion of rIL-2 systemically into humans have recently begun."

Without fear, of course, courage is only foolishness. Robert Handelman had courage. He never ceased to fear and yet he did not allow it to control him.

When we met, he was twenty-seven years old, not working, and had spent his entire life living with his mother. When he was five, his father had abandoned the family for good, and his mother had taken care of him since. Oddly, one got the sense that only his disease had made him begin to feel any responsibility for himself.

From West Virginia, he had enjoyed perfect health until two

years earlier, when a burning chest pain and a cough began to bother him. He went to the emergency room of the local hospital, where a doctor diagnosed his problem as an allergy, gave him an antihistamine, and sent him home. But he kept coughing.

Two months later, a mass appeared in his neck. In May 1982, he came to NIH with his mother. Unfortunately, Mr. Handelman had an aggressive liposarcoma, a rare cancer of the fatty tissue.

The emergency room doctor was not at fault. Seventy million Americans have a cough every year. Perhaps 200 have Mr. Handelman's type of cancer, and it does not show up on a routine X ray. There was no reason to suspect cancer or to run sophisticated tests, and a diagnosis made two months earlier would almost surely have made no difference anyway.

We resected the mass in his neck and gave him chemotherapy. Four months later we saw a shadow in the lung on an X ray. We operated again. It was benign. But Mr. Handelman's luck lasted only a few weeks. The mass reappeared on both sides of his neck and began to extend down into the mediastinum, the upper chest.

He received radiation therapy to shrink the tumor. In October, Liz Grimm's husband, Jack Roth, our chief thoracic surgeon, operated. He found the tumor wrapped around the aorta. It was unresectable, and he closed.

There was nothing any of us could offer Mr. Handelman anymore.

He understood his prognosis. He had an inoperable cancer that would surely kill him. It terrified him. Even compared to others in his situation, he was unusually anxious and depressed. The nurses taught him relaxation techniques. He saw a psychiatrist. He wanted to learn imaging, in which the patient visualizes his or her white blood cells devouring cancer cells. If a patient feels imaging or something else can help defeat the cancer and this helps the patient feel better, I encourage the patient to pursue these things—even though I do not believe they have any physical effect—so long as they do not interfere with effective treatment.

Yet for all his terror in the face of his disease, Mr. Handelman began to strive, to struggle not with his disease but with his life. Not long after his final operation, he met a girl, fell in love, and for the first time in his life moved out of his mother's home and in with the girl. In a strange way, moving out allowed him to feel good about both life in general and even his own life. I think it was a declaration to the world—and to himself—that he was still alive and that, although I sensed he had begun to lose hope, he wanted to fight.

When I told Mr. Handelman we had a new therapy involving recombinant IL-2, he eagerly agreed to try it. Whether courage comes from desperation or not, there was courage in this. I told him no one had ever given this material to a person before. I told him we wanted to push him hard, very hard, to find out the limits of the body's tolerance of this material. For the first time we had enough IL-2 to do this. And I told him that we knew IL-2 itself killed mice when they were given too much.

Most patients want to try any therapy that might help, no matter how risky. Some patients are extremely cautious, even while agreeing to try experimental therapies; each second of each day has value to them. They do not want to waste an instant, or lose one, and are concerned with safety above everything else.

Mr. Handelman was somewhere in between. He had fear and he also had a certain recklessness about him that went beyond just a desire to try anything that might work. It was as if risking his life made him more alive, as if testing the limits of his own fear made life more worth living, as if he felt he had done nothing in his life—but he would do this. We told him that he had absolute control over the treatment. At any time that he wanted us to stop, we would stop—instantly. With his face grim and drawn but also determined, he replied that he intended to tough this out no matter what the side effects were, and he would not ask us to stop. Clearly he meant it.

We admitted him on March 30, 1984, a Friday. He would become the first patient in our Phase I trial with rIL-2, which was designed to establish tolerated dosages. At 1:00 P.M. on Monday, April 2, we started his first dose of 720 units of rIL-2 per kilogram of bodyweight per hour, infused continuously over a twenty-four-hour period. Mike Lotze, nurse Claudia Seipp, and I stood at the foot of his bed. There was no need. We were giving him a tiny amount, even less than the first dose of Du Pont IL-2 we had given. He showed no side effects of any kind.

But the next day Mr. Handelman received 3,600 units per kilo per hour. His pulse quickened and his temperature rose to 38.9° Celsius, about 100° Fahrenheit.

We doubled the dose to 7,200 units per kilo per hour. He had fever, chills, and his platelet count dropped to half that of normal. For two days, we gave him that dosage. The weekend came and we gave him nothing; we let him rest for two days.

On Monday, April 9, he received 29,000 units per kilo per hour. It was the first time we had enough IL-2 to reach this dosage level. His fever rose to 40.1° Celsius—104.1° Fahrenheit—and his liver function became abnormal. He grew nauseated and lost his appetite. We gave him fluid to support him.

The next day he received the same dosage, then we dropped back to 7,200 units for three days.

We scanned his liver and spleen. The liver was enlarged and his hematocrit had dropped. We had to give him two units of blood.

Mr. Handelman's anxiety never left him. One could sense it in him the way he started whenever anyone entered his room, the way his eyes darted from one person to another as if seeking reassurance, the way he lay there silently but with his fists clenched. Yet his attitude had not changed since he began; he intended to tough this out and would not ask us to stop. We were inflicting constant nausea upon him, and racking nausea is one of the most debilitating and demoralizing symptoms a person can endure. Pain can often be easier to endure than nausea; only intense pain is harder. He remained anxious, and yet he complained little. Far from asking us to stop, he grimly wanted us to proceed.

The decision to press ahead was not his to make. He had the power to make us stop, but he could not tell us to go forward. That was our decision, a medical decision that it was still safe, and Mike and I discussed this constantly.

We gave him two days of rest, without any treatment. I was

reassured that his test results were moving toward normal even if they had not quite returned to normal.

We then began treatment again, administering 3,000 units per kilo per hour. Abnormal liver function returned.

I grew nervous. Although his liver function had seemed to recover during his brief rest, there was no way of knowing whether we were permanently damaging the liver, or whether other problems from side effects we had not yet seen could suddenly erupt.

At the same time, Mr. Handelman was in an absolutely dire situation because of his disease. It would certainly kill him soon unless the rIL-2 had some effect; treating him was not like treating a healthy volunteer.

And so on April 19, we decided to push further, to seek a limit. I knew how much IL-2 mice could tolerate in proportion to their body weight and we had not approached that figure. We raised the dosage to 72,000 units per kilo per hour for twenty-four hours, a rate of approximately 135 million units a day. This amount approximately equaled the entire first shipment of Du Pont IL-2, a supply with which we had treated a half-dozen patients with dosages stretched over weeks.

At 10:50 A.M. the next day, April 20, I was deeply concerned. His fever was 40.5° C—104.5° F. His blood clotting was abnormal. His liver enzymes were ten times normal.

I feared we were killing him.

We backed off.

Rapidly all his metabolic functions returned to normal. This was an enormous relief. A few days later he was discharged.

Mr. Handelman taught us much. Investigators had speculated that because the body itself produced IL-2, it would not cause any serious toxicity or side effects. Clearly that speculation was wrong. In large enough doses, IL-2 could kill. We also learned that the body did have a limit to the amount of IL-2 it would tolerate, and that tolerance was forty-fold less than mice in proportion to body weight. And we had reason to believe, although we did not know for certain, that the side effects disappeared after treatment stopped.

But one month later, at a follow-up visit, we saw no decrease in his tumors. A few months later Mr. Handelman died.

Until now, we had not had enough IL-2 to see side effects. Treating patients then was easy. Treating patients with the unlimited supplies of the rIL-2 had already become difficult. Now we were seeing side effects, and severe ones. It is very difficult as a doctor to inflict pain on a patient. It is much more difficult when one does not know if the treatment will do any good. I was torn between wanting to treat more patients, wanting to push each one to the limit of tolerance, and wanting to stop causing senseless agony.

We were raising hopes, subjecting patients to dangerous and extremely uncomfortable side effects, separating them from their home and families—at NIH patients come from all over the country and are often isolated from their families—and keeping them in the hospital with tubes stuck in their bodies in what could be the last days of their lives. We were stealing time from our patients, and time was their most precious possession.

And for what? I had now seen thirty straight deaths.

All these years critics had insisted that, even if immunotherapy could work in animal models, it would not work in man. Perhaps they were right.

Thirty straight deaths. I had known, and known well, each of those patients. Our interactions had been continuous and often intimate. In not a single instance had I seen any indication either of shrinkage of a tumor or of any other benefit. And now, the treatment I was giving inflicted additional suffering. My feelings shifted back and forth, between an expectation that the next patient would show a response and an increasing and corrosive fear that none ever would.

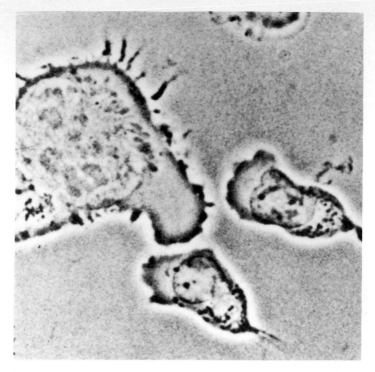

The top photograph shows a microscopic view of mouse T cells attacking a cancer cell (the largest of the cells). John R. Yannelli

Below, human T lymphocytes growing in IL-2, as seen under a scanning electron microscope. Cellco, Inc., Germantown, MD

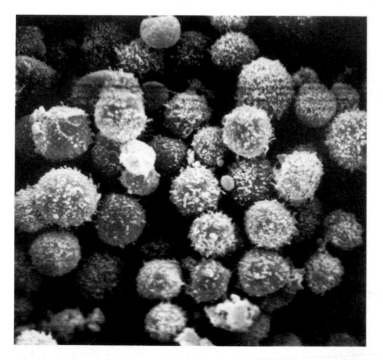

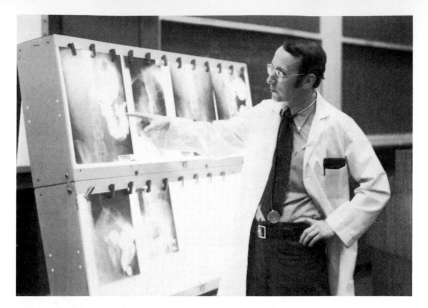

As a surgical resident at the Peter Bent Brigham Hospital in 1968, I met Mr. DeAngelo and learned of the spontaneous regression of his cancer; this was one of the factors that led to my search for an immune response to the disease.

In 1976, two years after I came to NIH as chief of surgery, we had a family get-together: my sister, Florence, my brother, Jerry, and I are behind my mother, Harriet, and father, Abraham.

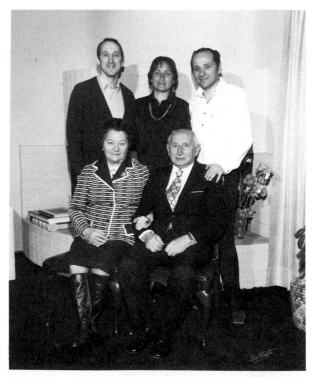

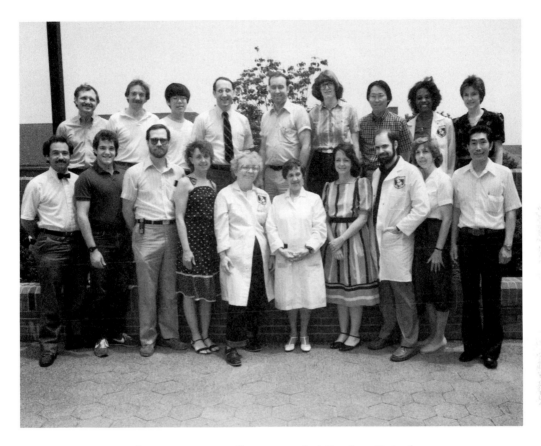

My research team in 1982: (front row, l-r) Stephen Ettinghausen, M.D., Evan Blonder, Anthony Raynor, M.D., Susan Schwarz, Cornelia Hyatt, Hilda Wexler, Deborah Wilson, Maury Rosenstein, Ph.D., Claudia Seipp, Suyu Shu, Ph.D.; (back row, l-r) Michael Lotze, M.D., James Mulé, Ph.D., Donald Tsai, myself, Paul Speiss, Lesley Frana, Alfred Chang, M.D., Yvette Matory, M.D., Elizabeth Grimm, Ph.D. William Branson

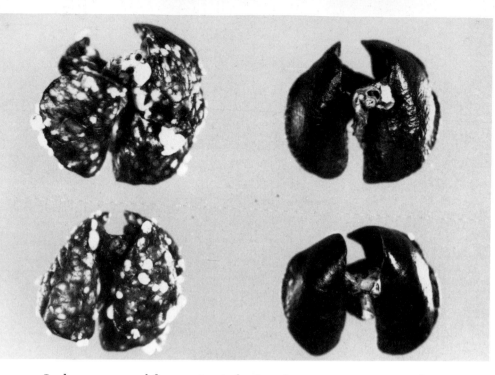

In lungs removed from untreated mice, the cancer appears as white nodules on a black background (because India ink has been injected into the trachea to make it easier to count the metastases). On the right, the mice have been treated with LAK cells and IL-2 and show almost no cancer. These types of animal experiments preceded our clinical trials with LAK cells and IL-2 in humans.

These chest X rays show the extensive spread of melanoma to the patient's lungs prior to treatment (left). The disappearance of the cancer following treatment with high-dose IL-2 alone is shown on the right. This was one of the first patients to exhibit cancer regression when treated with IL-2.

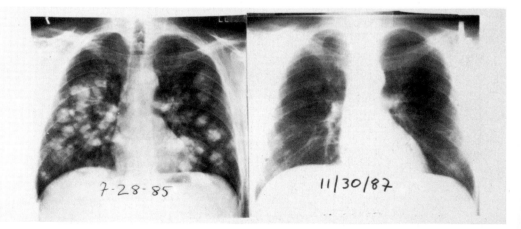

7-28-85   11/30/87

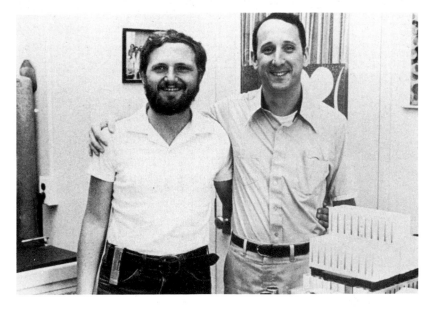

Mike Lotze and me in 1980. Mike, who was an important member of my research team, has recently moved to the University of Pittsburgh. William Branson

Jim Mulé is a key scientist in our current immunotherapy and gene therapy efforts. William Branson

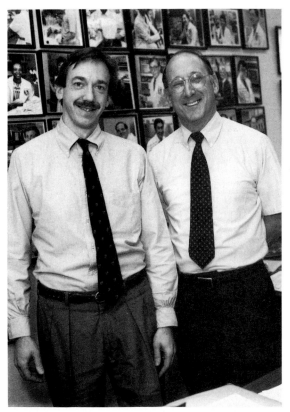

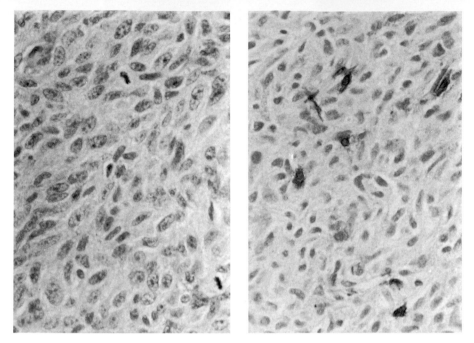

A microscopic view of the melanoma of Edwina Schreiber, one of
the first patients to receive gene-modified lymphocytes. In the
upper left, prior to treatment, the cancer cells fill the slide; in the
upper right and lower left, three and five days after treatment with
gene-modified lymphocytes and IL-2, the lymphocytes (the darker
cells) begin to attack the cancer. The slide on the lower right,
nineteen days after treatment, shows the lymphocytes
overwhelming the cancer.

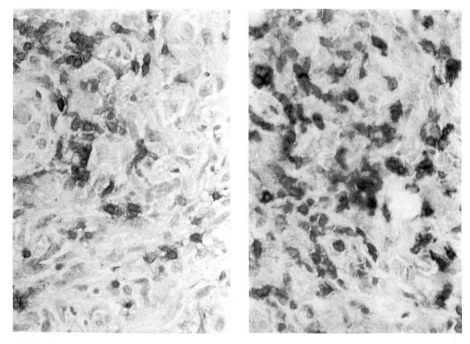

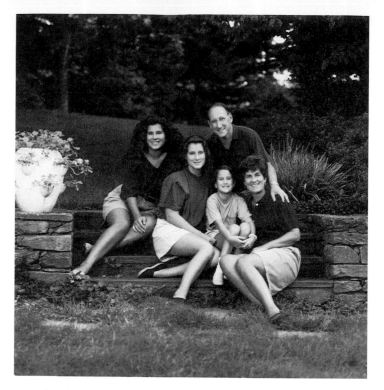

A 1990 family portrait: Here I am with (l-r) Beth, Rachel, Naomi, and Alice. Monte & Associates, Silver Spring, MD

As the first gene therapy experiments in humans were being planned in 1988, I conferred in the lab with my colleagues French Anderson and Michael Blaese. William Branson

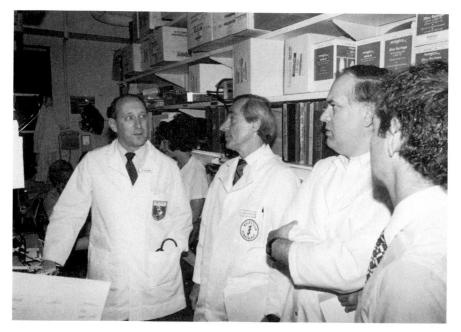

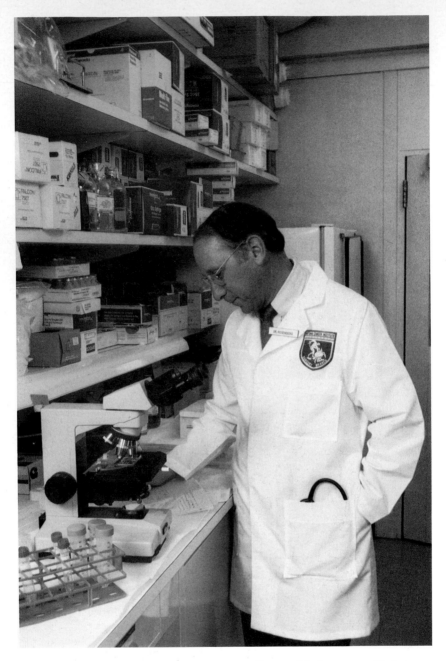

In the lab, 1992. The ability to genetically modify human cells has opened extraordinary possibilities for the development of new cancer treatments. Dennis Brack/Black Star

CHAPTER FIFTEEN

In the spring of 1984, for the first time in my life, a part of me wanted to get away. The cycle of hope, disappointment, and finally death that the patients receiving IL-2 went through was wearing me down and eroding my confidence. Perhaps for the first time at least a part of me began to doubt the path I had chosen to follow. I neither showed nor expressed this doubt to anyone in the lab, even while the burden of maintaining my own enthusiasm and everyone else's weighed increasingly upon me.

As a result, I again found it more and more difficult to leave the hospital, to leave my patients, to go home, even as day after day of death mocked my power to do anything for them. It seemed that only being in the hospital brought me comfort, while absence from it was disquieting to me. At the same time, I felt more and more a desire to escape completely.

Years before, during the brief gap between finishing my internship and starting graduate school, Alice and I drove across the country and camped out. We shared some of our closest times on this trip, and it has become one of our favorite memories.

It had always been understood between us that at some point we would take a similar trip with our children. Our oldest daughter, Beth, was then twelve. In a year or two she would no longer want to come with us on such a trip. Rachel was ten, old enough to enjoy it. Naomi was only two, too young to appreciate what she saw, but Alice and I felt we could do something else with her when she was older. I was anxious to spend more time with Alice and my daughters and realized this was likely to happen only if we were far from Bethesda.

Alice had never before urged me to get away from my work for more than a weekend. But she knew how I felt, knew I needed some respite, and reminded me of our plans to travel with our children.

Both the lab and the clinic were running smoothly. Al Baker was absolutely capable of handling the general administrative and clinical responsibilities of the branch. I had total confidence in Mike Lotze. He was absolutely capable of running the Phase I trial with rIL-2. Jim Mulé could handle the day-to-day research activities in my lab. Everything in the lab and the clinic was on as close to autopilot as it would ever be.

If ever there was a time for a trip around the country, this was that time.

I decided to take six weeks off as soon as my daughters got out of school. It was not the only manifestation of my discouragement, of my desire to escape.

My interest had always been combining science and medicine. I had stayed at NIH because the resources and atmosphere there were unlike anywhere else in the world. The numbers of excellent scientists and clinicians on campus and the possibilities generated by interactions with them create a critical mass that makes the National Institutes of Health the best of all biomedical research institutions.

For this reason I had always felt that I wanted to stay forever. Over the years several university posts had been offered to me. I always declined them instantly.

But in May 1984, the dean at The Johns Hopkins University School of Medicine inquired about my interest in the Halsted chair as professor and chairman of the Department of Surgery. The Halsted chair is probably the most prestigious surgical professorship in the world, and Hopkins is my alma mater. For the first time in my life, I agreed to consider a position outside NIH. I told myself that I was not serious about it, that I would not leave, but I visited the campus and listened to senior officials at the university.

At the same time, I decided to press NCI administrators to expand my lab. I wanted more space and people, along with money to support them. I had begun my investigations into T cells and IL-2 in 1977 with only Sue, Paul, and myself. By now, in 1984, I was working on immunotherapy along with two tenured senior investigators, Mike Lotze and Fred Chang, several more junior investigators, including both surgical fellows and postdoctoral Ph.D.s, and additional technicians. But investigators and technicians were overburdened and cramped; one person would be working on a mouse experiment on one lab bench, another on human studies on the adjacent bench, while a third at the next hood would be preparing LAK cells for patients. I wanted space for a new laboratory specifically devoted to producing cells for patients, and four technicians dedicated to only this task. We also needed a $500,000 machine that analyzed 50,000 cells a minute and the computers and personnel to support it. This would mark a major gearing up of my effort and would involve hiring more scientists as well. A comparable expansion of clinical resources for patients would probably follow: An entire team would be created to care for immunotherapy patients.

If it seemed an odd time to push for expansion, considering the devastating failure of every clinical therapy we had ever tried, if part of myself had even come to doubt my path, I still believed we were on the verge of important findings that could help cancer patients. I needed the additional resources to pursue them.

There may have been something deeper in my psyche that made me choose this moment to push for more resources. My reaction to failure has always been to work harder. So I pressed for the opportunity to work more intensively and harder.

In a muted confrontation, I told Vince DeVita, the director of NCI and a friend (we had coauthored a textbook on cancer with Sam Hellman, then chief of radiation therapy at Harvard), about both the inquiry from Hopkins and my desire for more space. Vince is well built, dark, charismatic, and totally self-assured; he is also highly intelligent and intuitive—his intuition supported by a well of knowledge about cancer greater than that of anyone I have known. He actively wants to make decisions, and as director controlled the single greatest source of biomedical research funds in the world. Today NCI spends approximately $1.6 billion a year; most of this money is disbursed in competitive grants to scientists in university labs, but a director has considerable discretionary power.

Vince had a reputation for aggressively using his power to advance programs he thought were promising, but when pushed, he was more likely to lash out than yield. Mentioning the Hopkins position while making a request was pushing him. But what mattered more than our little dance over the inquiry from Hopkins were my laboratory findings. I showed him the results that I considered powerful and even dramatic. They had not yet been published in *Science*, and they included photographs of the lungs of mice. Untreated mice had lungs thick with tumor; treated mice had clear, healthy lungs—their cancers had disappeared.

I presented a stronger case than I myself believed. To Vince, I did not express my doubts. He knew the problems anyway. Critics of immunotherapy had not been silent. Many things work in animals and fail in man. Many things. How well I knew that. He did not give me an answer about more space.

The day before leaving on my trip, I told Vince I was withdrawing my name from consideration for the position at Hopkins. It was inappropriate to continue to link my request for resources with this job inquiry. I repeated my arguments for more space and more people. Again Vince did not give me an answer.

In mid-June 1984, in a rented twenty-seven-foot-long RV, Alice, her mother, the children, and I began an 8,000-mile journey through the United States. I called the lab at most twice a week. For me to be out of touch like that was itself a jolt.

I did almost all the driving and it gave me time to think. The road seemed endless. The horizon never seemed to change; we could never reach it. And yet we made progress. There was something reassuring to me in that fact. But the distance I was traveling from NIH did not really hit me until we arrived at the Grand Canyon.

There is a peacefulness in observing and trying to understand something immense that one has no ability to affect or change. Astronomy makes me feel this way, and I am an amateur astronomer. One's impotence in the face of such immense magnitude is both humbling and relaxing.

The Grand Canyon must be the most spectacular sight on the planet. It is certainly the most spectacular sight *I* have ever witnessed. The beauty of its colors and my sense of the enormous natural forces that carved it moved me.

I literally spent hours sitting on the edge of the canyon, staring down into it. I could not see the bottom. Its magnificence overwhelmed me. The power of nature overwhelmed me. It drove me inward, into myself, and humbled me.

It also created in me a sense of wonder—wonder not only in the sense of awe or marveling, but also in the sense of trying to puzzle something out. Natural beauty opens my mind, makes me think grander thoughts. To witness something that seems incomprehensible and know that it exists is a reality so powerful that it forces me to confront other realities. And it makes me feel powerful myself, and determined to do powerful things.

Looking deep into the canyon, I could feel strength flowing into me, and it left me determined to do something important. It was the first of many such experiences on the trip.

Hour after hour on the road, while my children played or argued or sat silently as the miles passed, I thought about my work, thought through one idea after another in my mind. More than ever, I wanted to make progress and yet could find no way out of our stalemate. In my mind I reexamined every avenue the lab had explored in the past several years, searching for something we had missed, turning experiments inside out, searching for some new approach. It became frustrating; an idea for an experiment would come to me and I could not do it immediately.

There were also times—when hiking, or having dinner with my family around a campfire, or searching for galaxies through my telescope with my daughters on a clear dark night high in the mountains—that I felt totally detached from my life in Bethesda. I achieved a tense peace, a balance between enjoying the beauty and my family, and feeling anxiety and desperation over my separation from my work each time I called the lab. But as the end of the trip neared, I increasingly felt I had had enough. I needed to get back.

I returned to more disappointments. I began immediately to pursue what I considered the best idea that had occurred to me on the trip: to attach antibodies to LAK cells to increase their specificity and target them to tumors. After spending a year learning how to attach antibodies to a LAK cell and have the cell maintain its killing activity, Avi Eisenthal and I finally gave these altered cells to animals. They had no effect on the animals' tumors and we abandoned the approach.

But there was more immediately discouraging news. I was especially close to the fourth patient to receive recombinant IL-2, Susan Robidoux; when I think of her my pulse still races a little. I think particularly of what was probably the most difficult operation I have ever performed.

We met when she was thirty-five, two years earlier. She was then in another experimental protocol at NCI and was operated on. Her colon was removed, and a metastasis was seen on her liver but left untouched. Six lymph nodes were also removed; three were positive. It was a very aggressive cancer. Three weeks after the operation she came to see me.

The lesion in the liver was near the vena cava, the major vein in the body. This made an operation to remove it life-threatening, but removing it would give her a chance—a very small one—of being cured of her disease. She was young, with young children, and otherwise healthy. I thought the chance of a cure made the operation worth the risk. Without it she was likely to live no longer than six months. Neither chemotherapy nor radiation therapy would have prolonged her life. I discussed this with her and her husband, recommended the operation, and together we decided to proceed only if no metastases were found at any site other than the liver.

I began the surgery with a large midline incision from her pubis to her xiphoid, opening her entire abdomen. Good exposure is key to safe surgery. I noted an ovarian cyst and biopsied it. It was negative. The periaortic lymph nodes were negative. With my fingers I felt the liver itself. On the left lobe there were two clearly cancerous lesions: one 6 centimeters in diameter, which we already knew about, but there was also one 2 centimeters wide. My fingers felt the right lobe and found another small abnormality. I biopsied it. It was not cancer. All her disease seemed confined to the left lobe of her liver. The tumor rested directly on the left hepatic vein and the vena cava. Bleeding from a large vein is the most difficult to control. Blood spurts out of arteries, making it easy to find and isolate the problem, but veins are soft and blood wells up out of them. Gaining access to this particular vein is very difficult, making it particularly hard to control bleeding. The risk of proceeding was great, but she did have a real chance of being cured if we could remove the lesions.

I decided to push ahead.

I tied off the blood vessels at the base of the liver but the tumor occluded my view of the back of the liver, so I extended the incision into her left chest to increase the exposure of the hepatic veins and the vena cava. Then I started separating the two lobes of the liver. Deep in the liver the cancer extended into the right lobe. We had to increase the amount of liver we would remove. Liver tissue is very soft, and blood vessels are embedded deeply in it. As we removed the left lobe, major hemorrhaging occurred.

There are eight units of blood in the body. Very quickly Mrs. Robidoux ran through ten units while we struggled to gain control.

We were now six hours into the operation. I was suturing, putting clips on blood vessels, packing Avitene, Gelfoam, and thrombin—all designed to control bleeding—against the raw liver edge and was making little progress. Blood continued to well up.

We were losing ground. The more I sutured and clipped, the more the liver bled.

Everyone in the O.R. grew frantic—we all became more crisp, more intense, more concentrated, as if we believed our combined focused wills could affect Mrs. Robidoux's body. But I was losing control of the case. I could feel her slipping away. We were losing her and I was running out of ideas about how to stop the bleeding. For only the second or third time in my life, I decided I had to leave the O.R. to regroup.

I carefully packed gauze pads tightly against the liver and all of the raw bleeding areas, and positioned both of the resident's hands against them and told him to press tightly. As long as pressure was applied, the bleeding would be controlled. She would remain stable. I told the resident and nurses I would be in the doctors' lounge a few steps away. And I walked out.

I sat down alone in the lounge, leaned back, and inhaled deeply, trying to think, trying to collect myself. For fifteen minutes I sat there, rising only to get some apple juice from the nurses' refrigerator. I had no new ideas. There were no subtleties here, at least none that I could see. But I did freshen myself. I closed my eyes, took a few more deep breaths, and returned to the O.R. My fingers moved with a restored purpose, attacking one bleeding vessel at a time. One after another, I sutured or clipped them. And the pressure the resident had applied helped, while the earlier suturing and clipping seemed finally to be having some effect. Things started to work. I still could not stop the bleeding entirely but left drains in and closed at 5:45 P.M. We had begun the operation at 9:30 A.M.

Mrs. Robidoux lost a total of nineteen units of blood. At 6:00 I saw her husband and told him that I was concerned she might not survive the operation. I vividly recall speaking to him in the waiting area down a long corridor from the O.R. For more than eight hours, knowing that this was a dangerous operation, he had been frantic and now he became distraught. He started to talk about what she meant to him and to their children. I had nothing to offer him except some hope.

She needed two more units of blood but then stabilized and

recovered well. Fourteen days after the operation she was discharged. She had pushed us to allow her to get home in time to take her oldest child to the first day of kindergarten.

Every time I saw her in follow-up, my belly writhed as I relived the terror of her operation. I hoped that for once the odds might go her way, but they did not. Her cancer returned. She failed chemotherapy.

In April 1984, two months before I began my trip around the country with my family, we finally offered her rIL-2. We pushed her as high as 72,000 units per kilogram of body weight per hour for five days. We thought it was a huge dosage. Mr. Handelman had received that dosage for only one day.

She, too, had a difficult time with treatment, developing an infection at the site of infusion. She suffered other side effects as well. I thought surely if the rIL-2 worked at all, she stood a chance of responding.

She completed her rIL-2 treatment before I left on my trip and had her first post-treatment follow-up visit while I was on it. In a small roadside phone booth in Wyoming, I learned that her cancer had not responded. The report made me want to return to the hospital immediately but I could not leave my family.

When I did return, I was greeted with information about other patient failures. It mocked all the grand thoughts I had had while sitting at the edge of the Grand Canyon.

The only good news was that during my absence DeVita had walked through all the Surgery Branch space with Al Baker and decided to give me more resources. While gratifying, his decision did not seem cause for celebration. I wondered how much the subtext of my request—my mention of the Hopkins inquiry—had influenced him, and whether he was simply trying to keep me content. Besides, the federal bureaucracy moves slowly. Although preliminary signs of work appeared—a carpenter would show up and measure something, or a coil of wire would suddenly appear in the corridor and then disappear—I expected it to take months, possibly a year or even more, before my lab actually got more space and additional personnel. And given the results from our clinical trials, given the prognosis of Susan Robidoux, I was not in a mood to celebrate anything. I was only in the mood to work harder.

On a Saturday night a few weeks after my return, I worked most of the day and went home for dinner. I was restless. Alice and the kids went to bed. I tried to sleep but could not and read scientific journals for a while. The restlessness continued. Reading did not comfort me. Finally I decided to return to the lab.

It was late, after midnight, and, with almost the entire route from my home to NIH through residential neighborhoods, the road was empty. The NIH campus was similarly deserted. I parked. The sound of the car door closing, of my key clicking in the lock, seemed to echo through the cavernous garage. Through the night, all night, one routinely sees investigators on their way to or from monitoring an experiment. The whole building had an empty, even eerie, feel.

But as I climbed the stairs, strange noises came to me. One sounded like a hammer exploding on wood. It was a noise that did not belong, but still it sounded strong and confident, repetitive and sure-handed, so much so that despite its strangeness it was reassuring. Clearly it came from a carpenter who knew his business. Then the unmistakable buzzing roar of a power saw erupted, drowning out the hammer. A few more steps and I opened the stairwell door by my lab. Suddenly confronting me was a burst of bustle—more hammering, another power saw, a corridor choked with lumber, tables, scientific equipment, and half a dozen men in hard hats moving amid a blaze of lights and sound.

The contrast between this hive of activity and the emptiness of the night stunned me for an instant, as if I had happened upon an entirely different world, but the explanation was obvious.

The workers moving about in the corridor were remodeling labs which had belonged to Alan Rabson, the director of a major division of NCI. Now the space would be part of my lab.

On direct orders from DeVita—it could happen no other way—these laboratories were being built at a pace I did not believe was possible in the government. Perhaps to have found these men here seems a small thing to someone who does not know the effort required to move the bureaucracy. But I did know. DeVita had exerted enough effort to compress what normally took as long as a year down to a few weeks and days. He had exerted himself enough to get men working in the middle of the night on a Saturday, working with a haste and urgency I had never before seen in all my years at NIH, working at the price of disrupting all the budgets and schedules and regulations according to which the federal bureaucracy normally moves, working at the price of disrupting DeVita's and perhaps my own relationship with Rabson.

I had put almost ten years of my life directly into the effort of developing immunotherapy, and indirectly more than double that many years. In all that time, not a single person outside my own laboratory had ever done more than express interest in what we were doing. Critics had never ceased arguing that it was quite possible that immunotherapy could not work in man. But these workers moving in the corridor demonstrated that someone outside my own laboratory believed as I believed. Now DeVita was putting himself on the line next to me. I felt isolated no more. For the first time in all the years I had pursued this idea, I had a sense of history. I had as yet seen only death. I had observed no hint of a response in any patient yet. But I felt isolated no more.

I thought, *Maybe I can really do this thing.* Standing there outside my expanding laboratory, shading my eyes from the otherworldly brilliance of the magnesium torch, excusing myself to the workers moving around me—they no doubt wondering who this man was with this bizarre, quasi-mystical look on his face— silent, for this one moment, hating the disease and wanting to kill it, I allowed myself to think, *Yes. I can do this thing. Yes.*

I continued to give patients recombinant IL-2. They continued to die. One after another, their cancers failed to respond.

I had experimented with adoptive immunotherapy in seventy-five patients through the years. My efforts had been flailing and futile. The first six had received pig lymphocytes. Three had received small numbers of lymphocytes grown in our primitive IL-2. Twenty-seven had received the nonspecific killer cells. Sixteen had received Du Pont's purified natural IL-2. Now twenty-three had received recombinant IL-2 in, I thought, large doses. All had died, or would soon die. None showed any sign of having benefited from the therapy; many had suffered through debilitating side effects.

I had gotten to know all of them, all of them had looked to me expectantly—confident that I had it in my power to cure them—and my efforts had failed each of them. Cumulatively their names were almost too much to bear, like visiting the Vietnam Memorial. Linda Karpaulis. Nelson Edwards. Susan Robidoux. Sheila Hopeland. Amanda Pritchard. Robert Handelman. Raul Fernandez. Tom Showard.

But I still had not tried the one therapy that worked consistently in the animal models—a combination of LAK cells and recombinant IL-2.

The FDA had not allowed us to treat patients with this combination. Regulators insisted that we needed to know more about each element individually before combining them. Now we did know more.

LAK cells grown in rIL-2 behaved like the other killer cells we had given. Their chief side effect was fever and chills, and they seemed by themselves quite safe. If we gave enough rIL-2, we now knew, it was highly toxic. The toxicity was dose-related; it increased as the dose increased. Weight gain—of up to forty pounds over a period of days—was the most common side effect and could be dangerous. The weight increase occurred because fluid leaked into tissues of the body; this fluid had the potential to fill the lungs and suffocate the patient. There were other side effects on circulating white cells, the liver, and the kidneys. These side effects appeared to be transient; they appeared to end when the treatment ended.

I submitted everything we had learned from our clinical trials to the FDA and asked for permission to give LAK cells and rIL-2 in combination.

The agency approved this combined therapy on October 4,

1984. Within one or two days after receiving permission, I treated the first patient with the combined therapy and soon treated three more. But I was cautious and began with low dosages of IL-2 given by continuous infusion.

Strangely, all my other therapies I had begun with optimism, but not this one. Even as I started this therapy, I did not have a good feeling about my approach.

It seemed futile to me to administer it in a cautious and conservative way. Yet I was being cautious and conservative. I felt it was vital to be aggressive in order to get a response. Yet I was not being aggressive.

Perhaps I was afraid to be aggressive. Always before, any therapy I had tried lagged behind some promising experimental result. Always before, there had been reason to believe that even if the therapy failed we would learn much from it to help us in the future. Always before, there had been the promise that some new information about to be uncovered in the lab would explain and correct our failures in the clinic.

But now this combination of LAK cells and IL-2 was all I had to offer. If it did not work, I had no place else to go. I had no other therapy to try, nor any experiments indicating a new path to follow.

If aggressive treatment failed, all our years of effort might be for nothing. I had published almost 250 scientific papers by then, the overwhelming majority dealing with immunotherapy. We had made what I considered important scientific observations, but there would be little satisfaction in this for me if the information did not lead to new treatments. If that were the case, then all that I had done would be, to me, a failure, all my efforts a fool's errand. I would have to start all over in the laboratory. Perhaps I was not treating the patients aggressively because I feared confronting this reality.

I recalled my thoughts about Mr. DeAngelo that time we met, back in 1968 in the veterans' hospital in West Roxbury, Massachusetts, and his sardonic look, his look that said he understood the ironies of life and had even had the better of those ironies. Mr. DeAngelo would have had the last laugh after all.

195

Thinking of all this, I grew tired of being conservative, weary of it, and my weariness overcame any timidity. Even before follow-up appointments were made to evaluate the effect of the combined therapy on the first four patients—none would respond—I decided I had had enough.

There is a saying of a famous Hasidic rabbi, Rabbi Nachman of Bratzslav, which I learned as a boy: "It is forbidden to despair."

I did not despair, but out of desperation came hope. The best information we had came from the animal models, and I would follow them exactly.

The animals that responded had received three bolus injections of IL-2 a day, along with LAK cells. I had not given IL-2 in this manner to a single patient. I had chosen not to because the animals had gotten the injections intraperitoneally, into the abdomen. When given that way, the IL-2 was released slowly into the bloodstream. I thought that giving a patient IL-2 by continuous intravenous infusion over twenty-four hours most closely resembled the animal model.

But even an intraperitoneal injection sent a sudden rush of IL-2 through the animal's circulatory system. Continuous infusion of IL-2 did not provide patients with this rush. I had wanted to protect them from it, but perhaps it was necessary.

I decided that the next patient would be treated as the animals were. I would give the next patient large numbers of LAK cells and a high dose of IL-2 by bolus injection three times a day. The injections would be administered intravenously, which made the treatment even more aggressive than that used in the animal models.

The next patient was Linda Granger. Nothing would ever be the same again.

PART FOUR

THE END OF
THE BEGINNING

CHAPTER SIXTEEN

Linda Granger had long straight hair and was very neat, but she did not seem to pay a lot of attention to her appearance. This may have been a manifestation of her self-confidence. One got a sense of strength from her.

Her father had spent his career in the Air Force and she had joined the Navy after college. When I first met her she was thirty-three years old and had spent her adult life as a Navy officer doing jobs that in earlier generations had been done by men. She approached things in terms of solving a problem, avoided small talk, and rarely dwelled on a subject in conversation or explored feelings. Although quiet and serious whenever she talked with me, she also seemed to be someone who could indulge herself if she chose to. Her goal, she once said, was to make admiral. She was straightforward, the kind of person who wanted to hear the truth straight.

And she always remained in control of herself—perhaps too much so. Although she seemed close to her family, she always came to the hospital alone. This was unusual. Once she explained, "I don't reach out when I'm in trouble. I focus on the problem. When the problem is so large, I redirect my energy. I circle the wagons. My family never came with me to the hospital because I didn't want to have to worry about them, too. Depend on thyself."

Her attitude was such that I could almost believe her problem did not terrify her. I knew better. She had to be terrified. Bravado was her defense, but at the same time her courage was real. I saw her cry once, and it was very unlike her; her tears came long after her experience, when she was recounting it and the immensity of what she had endured struck her. She never cried during her treatment.

In 1982 a mole, which she had always had on her right scapula, began, in her words, "to bubble over." It was removed at Bethesda Naval Hospital, a massive facility directly across Wisconsin Avenue from NIH, and diagnosed as melanoma. Her lymph nodes were all negative, but the lesion was 2.7 millimeters thick—very thick. Based on that, her doctor told her she had a 50 percent chance of a recurrence. A year passed without one, and her doctor told her there was now a 75 percent chance that she had been cured. She was thrilled and, a lieutenant commander, took a new post in Guam in November 1983, as the Flag Secretary, a job she defines as "sitting on an admiral's staff keeping the paper going and looking important."

But within a few weeks after starting this job she began to feel small, hard, marblelike bumps under her skin. One was biopsied. The melanoma had returned. She was given the choice of several hospitals to go to and chose one in Biloxi, Mississippi, because it was closest to her parents, then in Pensacola, Florida. But Biloxi was Air Force territory. The admiral she worked for believed she would get better treatment at Bethesda. He overrode her request and sent her there.

At Bethesda she was told she probably had three months to a year to live.

"It seemed unreal," she later said. "I felt fine. Something wasn't clicking in my head. After some more tests the doctor came back and said, 'Really good news. None of your internal organs are affected yet. You may have as long as seventeen months.' "

A doctor from NIH happened to accompany a Navy doctor on rounds, saw her, and suggested an experimental NIH protocol in Frederick, Maryland. She sought it out, was accepted, and endured three separate experimental therapies, one with monoclonal antibodies, one with alpha-interferon administered intravenously, and one with alpha-interferon injected into the lesions.

Her cancer did not respond. Her tumors were growing and now numbered a dozen.

One doctor at the Frederick NIH facility said her disease would kill her. There was nothing else to do, he said. No chemotherapy has yet been developed that affects metastatic melanoma for any but the briefest intervals, and the side effects can destroy a patient's quality of life. He advised her to enjoy whatever time she had left, perhaps travel, go to Europe.

She thought going to Europe might make sense. The experimental therapies had been draining and she was tired of them, tired of the pain and tired of spending any of the precious remaining days in hospitals with tubes sticking into her arms. The idea of just accepting her fate, of resting, of living out her life peacefully was not unattractive to her, she later said. But another doctor mentioned my work and referred her to us. Her family pushed her to keep fighting, to explore this final possibility. She did.

Once she made this decision, she committed herself. In fact, she expressed something that worries many patients in experimental therapies—a fear that she would somehow not measure up to a doctor's expectations and be expelled from the program. She knew this was her last opportunity.

Her first appointment with us was on November 14, 1984, when we met. We discussed LAK and IL-2 therapy and she said she wanted it. On November 25, she was admitted.

I sat down with her and reviewed in detail all the laboratory data concerning our protocol, as well as the potential benefits and risks of the treatment. She just nodded. It seemed to me that she was going to do this no matter what I said. By now she had multiple melanoma nodules appearing on her back, buttocks, and extremities. I finished my explanation of the informed consent. She agreed to proceed.

Because of the unique side effects of the immunotherapy, I did not have the regular clinical staff treat patients receiving it. Steve Ettinghausen was taking care of Ms. Granger, with Claudia Seipp, the nurses on our 2 East ward, and myself.

Claudia was one of the first people I hired when I came to NIH. Almost all the nurses here are exceptional and accept a lower salary than area hospitals pay because they want to learn and help develop state-of-the-art medicine. Even within this group, Claudia stood out. By the time I arrived, she had worked at NIH for several years and had been head nurse in two different wards. She is intelligent and articulate, knows relevant facts, and thinks through their implications. But beyond any objective qualities, there is something very solid and reliable about her. She inspires confidence. She was capable of setting up and running a program, screening and following patients for our protocols, and making decisions. The Surgery Branch had never had a research nurse; I offered her a job as our first one. Routinely she accepts responsibilities that would make many nurses uncomfortable.

Claudia and Steve Ettinghausen worked particularly well together and became close friends. Steve wonders about things, thinks about them, turns them over and looks at them from different angles. Today, well into his thirties, he still describes himself as having "not yet found my niche"; before beginning surgical training he spent two years in internal medicine and one year training as a pathologist. I consider him accomplished—perhaps more accomplished than he thinks he is—and I recently convinced him to leave Sloan-Kettering in the middle of a fellowship and return to NIH as a senior investigator.

Back then, he was a surgical fellow and had finished his clinical rotation. Although he had started a lab project, I wanted him to monitor Linda Granger closely.

The day we admitted her, we also put a central line in, a minor surgical procedure to insert a large-bore catheter into the subclavian vein just below the collarbone. This gave us instant access to the bloodstream to both administer medication and enable us to measure the central venous pressure, an indicator of adequate blood volume. We also biopsied two lesions; the pathologist's report concluded that the disease was "metastatic malignant melanoma . . . Two specimens were similar, nearly completely viable."

But we did not know how best to coordinate pheresing her with administering IL-2. We needed to perform both procedures and yet the one interfered with the other. Phereses were necessary to obtain lymphocytes for us to transform into killer cells. Since we intended to give her LAK cells every few days for several weeks, she would have to undergo this procedure repeatedly. But IL-2 drives lymphocytes from the bloodstream; when IL-2 is given continuously, lymphocytes do not reappear for seven to ten days, at which time they rebound in much larger numbers. How could we make LAK cells if the phereses yielded no lymphocytes? To allay this problem somewhat, we decided to pherese her twice before giving her any IL-2. After that, we would repeat the procedure, get as many lymphocytes as we could while waiting for the rebound, and hope for the best.

On November 26, we pheresed her for the first time, then did it again on November 27. Each time she spent several hours with tubes diverting her entire blood flow through a machine, which used centrifugal force to separate her blood into its components, allowing us to remove lymphocytes before reinfusing it back into her body.

Murine LAK cells take three days of growth in culture to reach maximum killing efficiency. And I was going to treat Linda Granger exactly the way we treated mice.

So, three days after the first pheresis, when the LAK cells should have achieved their maximum ability to kill, the lab harvested the first dosage of killer cells, spinning them out of the culture and concentrating them in a standard plastic bag. As soon as the cells were ready for infusion, Claudia carried them to the ward.

At 2:40 P.M. on November 29, we gave Linda Granger her first LAK infusion of 3.4 billion cells. It took almost an hour for them to drip in. She suffered from chills. After the infusion she began receiving bolus intravenous injections every eight hours of 72,000 units of IL-2 per kilogram of body weight.

The next day we performed another pheresis and infused the second LAK dose, prepared from the November 27 pheresis. We also gave three more bolus injections of IL-2. Again, five minutes after the LAK infusion she had chills. We gave her meperidine to control them.

For six days this cycle continued of three doses of IL-2 a day, with LAK infusions and phereses every two or three days.

I saw her four or five times each day and Steve Ettinghausen, who was writing the actual medication orders, saw her more often and checked with me whenever any change in her status occurred.

At the end of the first week, having seen minimal side effects, I tripled the dose of IL-2. She now was getting 216,000 units per kilo three times day, a total of over 40 million units daily.

By December 10, Claudia's notes reported that Ms. Granger complained this treatment was rougher than the earlier experimental therapies she had tried, adding, "Patient very uncomfortable with side effects—edema, joint pain, mouth sores."

Ms. Granger could not eat, vomited often, felt too weak to get up from the bed or even talk to her family, and had difficulty breathing. She called it "the most difficult month of my life. You wonder, 'Why am I doing this? It isn't worth it.' It was also frightening. For the first time since everything began, I feared that I would not leave the hospital."

I talked the situation over with her and encouraged her to proceed. This was her final option. She agreed to continue.

On December 10, she got her seventh LAK infusion and two doses of IL-2, and then we backed off. We pheresed her the next day, but did not give her either cells or IL-2, then gave her a second day without treatment on December 11.

Even so, that same day she gained six kilos of body weight—more than thirteen pounds—in twenty-four hours. She had previously gained twenty-two pounds in the two weeks since we started the treatment. All of the weight gain—she had so far gone from 122 pounds to 157 pounds—came from the vast amounts of fluid she was retaining.

I was pushing her. I was going to go as far as I could and as far as she could. I was not going to hold anything back.

On December 13, we started the IL-2 again, although because of the weight gain I dropped it back to the 72,000-units-per-kilogram dosage. On December 14, she received her eighth LAK infusion and three doses of IL-2.

On December 16, Claudia noted, "She seems to be tolerating the IL-2 better now."

The IL-2 continued.

On Thursday, December 17, we gave her two more doses of IL-2 and at approximately 4:10 P.M. another LAK infusion, her ninth. I was pushing her very hard.

Every Thursday afternoon I have a lab meeting I call a "tea." One investigator presents his work in an amphitheater. To build camaraderie, I encourage everyone, including secretaries, to attend. Coffee and cookies are served first, then whoever is speaking usually shows slides for five minutes from some trip to an exotic or beautiful destination. After the trip slides, the secretaries leave and the scientific presentation begins.

I was already at tea. Steve Ettinghausen was checking the ward just before going to the tea himself. A nurse shouted to him and he ran over. At a glance he could tell this was serious and asked a nurse to get me at the conference, then a moment later sent another surgical fellow to get me.

Ms. Granger was ashen and cyanotic. Her skin had a blue cast, indicating severe oxygen depletion. She was struggling to breathe at forty times a minute, and her pulse was 140. Steve drew her blood gases, which later showed poor oxygenation.

He sat her up to ease her breathing. It did not ease. He gave her oxygen and aminophylline to dilate the airways in her lung, and he hoped she would get better. She did not get better. Now Steve faced a true crisis. He is thoughtful and even meditative. This moment demanded action.

But acting was complicated. The fellows left every clinical decision to me or, if they could not find me, Mike Lotze. They made almost no independent decisions about treating an immunotherapy patient.

Ms. Granger was not improving. He considered intubating her—putting her on a respiratory machine and having the machine breathe for her. In an experimental therapy, this is automatically defined as a Grade 4 Toxicity, a life-threatening situation. Steve worried that this would reflect poorly on the therapy. No immunotherapy patient had ever been intubated before. Partly for this reason, Steve later said, he hesitated to do so. Intubating a conscious patient can also be dangerous. But he was worried that he should have done so immediately.

Instead, he started to put in a nasal tracheal tube to further help her breathing. While he was doing this, she coughed up frothy fluid from severe pulmonary edema.

Then, suddenly, she stopped breathing.

Unconscious, she slumped backward. Her heart continued to beat but her pulse dropped to twenty beats a minute, a rate insufficient to sustain life. She was on the verge of death.

Instantly Steve intubated her, forcing the tube into her mouth and down her throat. Fluid gushed out of the tube—her lungs were full of water. He began cardiopulmonary resuscitation and injected atropine to increase her heart rate.

The messages had not yet reached me and I was still downstairs in the amphitheater for tea. In a dull relentless monotone over the hospital loudspeaker came the words, "Code Blue. 2 East . . . Code Blue. 2 East . . . Code Blue. 2 East . . ."

The moment I heard the Code Blue, I knew it had to be Linda Granger and I raced upstairs.

By the time I arrived she was surrounded by doctors and nurses. The tube was in her lungs and she was breathing 100 percent oxygen. Her blood pressure had recovered.

Steve did precisely the right thing. It took courage for him to act. He waited until it had to be done. The instant it had to be done, he did it. Otherwise, Linda Granger might well have died right then.

Linda regained consciousness as soon as the oxygen flow to her brain returned. She was given morphine and transferred to the ICU at 5:20 P.M., approximately forty-five minutes after her respiratory failure. We gave her massive doses of diuretics to help remove the excess fluid. She recovered quickly and was extubated the next day while we carefully monitored her ability to breathe on her own. The day after that she was transferred from the ICU back to the ward. We ended her IL-2 treatment.

It had been frightening for me as well as for her, but if combining LAK cells and IL-2 did not work against cancer, it was the end of these efforts. I had to find out if they held any promise at all. Everything was on the line. And so I had been determined not to stop pushing her until I was made to stop.

I was made to stop.

In three weeks she received many times the IL-2 that any previous patient had received, and billions of LAK cells. She was left with emotional scars. For months she continued to be terrified about not getting enough air and could sleep only when sitting up, supported by several pillows, with fans blowing air into her face. But her only physical scar was a chipped tooth from the laryngoscope used to insert the tube. We sent her to our dentist. We discharged her just in time to get home for Christmas, although she remained too weak to travel alone. A friend flew with her to her parents' home in Florida.

Her tumors showed no change.

On December 19, the day she returned to the ward from the ICU, we biopsied one of her lesions. The pathologist's report did not come back for several days. It was somewhat different from the report on her pretreatment biopsy, but usual lesion-to-lesion variation could account for the difference. Still, the report stated that the samples showed "metastatic melanoma and focal necrosis." Some of this tumor was necrotic—dead. The report also noted something curious: "Mild lymphocyte infiltration is present in the periphery of the lesion."

On January 9, 1985, Ms. Granger returned for her first follow-up appointment and Steve Ettinghausen measured the nodules. There was no change. We biopsied another lesion and asked her to return for another follow-up appointment in a month.

The pathologist's report on this biopsy was stranger: "Appearance . . . of tumor cell ghosts is consistent with patient's previously diagnosed malignant melanoma . . . Lymphocytes seen . . . No viable tumor is identified."

I asked Steve to call her and ask how she felt. He did. She felt fine, except for the fears about not breathing. She was thrilled to learn that this particular tumor seemed to be dead, but she had many tumors over much of her body and had not seen any change in them. If the tumors were really dying, they should be getting smaller and they were not.

Four days before this second biopsy was performed, on January 5, we began to treat our second patient.

I learned long ago that cancer presses upon families like weight on an arch. If the relationship is structurally sound, the disease can bind them more tightly together. But if there is a weakness or flaw in the structure, the relentless, unceasing pressure exerts such stress that the relationship implodes. Perhaps any extreme burden does this; I know that cancer does.

James Jensen was a troubled, even tormented, man who had endured illness almost his entire life. Tall, strong, well built, and attractive, a farmer from the rural South, he would sit stoically puffing on a pipe or chewing tobacco—and saying nothing. He kept much inside him.

At eighteen, after enduring many years of discomfort and occasional exquisite pain, a large cancer was found in his right colon. A surgeon removed the colon. A dozen years passed of good health, but in 1976 Mr. Jensen came to us with rectal cancer. His wife was with him. She was much shorter than he, attractive, and a nurse, and they had two young children. He entered a protocol and randomized to fulgerization, a procedure in which the surgeon, Al Baker, burned off the cancer with hot cautery. The alternative was far more extensive and morbid surgery.

Three years later a follow-up test showed that his CEA, a protein produced by cancer cells, had risen to twelve. His cancer had returned. X rays showed lesions in his liver and we resected three liver metastases. One year later, in 1980, the cancer returned in the rectum.

Treatment required the removal of his entire rectum, and a colostomy. A side effect was impotence. He was then thirty-six years old, extremely vital and good-looking, with a young and attractive wife. They had already gone through much together. Now they could no longer have intercourse. This clearly eroded his self-image and gnawed at him in other ways. In August 1981, a shadow appeared in his lung X rays on another follow-up visit; we operated and removed lung metastases. And he began to suspect his wife was having an affair, which she denied.

In September 1981, we gave him a penile implant, inserting two flexible rods into his penis, which created a permanent semi-erection and allowed him to have intercourse. It did not help their relationship. We offered counseling. This did not help either. And his disease was progressing.

In 1982, we removed multiple lung nodules. In June 1983, we removed more lung mets. In November the lung mets returned and he began several different chemotherapy regimens outside NIH. He responded to none. Apparently he continued to accuse his wife of having an affair. Their lives were hell, she told a nurse. The burden of his accusations, the combination of love and fear she felt, and the strain of the disease wore away at her.

She became distraught and moved in with her mother. Then she wanted to move back with him. He refused to take her back. He was a proud man, proud and stoic, and rage built in him. Meanwhile his lung lesions were growing. Finally husband and wife reconciled. Late in 1984, at approximately the time Linda Granger was going through her most difficult time, we offered him the LAK-IL-2 therapy. He accepted.

On January 3, 1985, we admitted him and the next day put in a subclavian line.

Because we had not seen shrinkage in Linda Granger's tumors, we treated him somewhat differently than we had treated her. We had pheresed her even while her lymphocyte population was depleted during the early IL-2 injections. We gave Mr. Jensen IL-2 alone for a prolonged period, then waited until the lymphocytes rebounded before trying to prepare LAK cells.

On January 5, we started him with 72,000 units of IL-2 per kilogram of body weight by bolus injection three times a day. On January 11, we tripled the dose. Side effects began—most worrisome were high fever and low blood pressure—and we canceled one dose of IL-2, but returned to three doses a day on January 12. On January 14, his lymphocyte counts rebounded to numbers high above normal. We stopped giving IL-2, then pheresed him five days in a row. Because of the phereses his platelet count dropped to 30,000, a dangerous level; normal is 250,000 to 400,000. His count was low enough that the slightest hemorrhage could lead to a major loss of blood. But we harvested a large number of cells.

On Friday, January 18, he received his first infusion of 8.9 billion LAK cells, followed by IL-2. The next day he received another 8.9 billion cells and two days later 12.4 billion cells, also along with IL-2. These were many more cells than Linda Granger received.

Then we stopped. We had used up the supply of his LAK cells. And he was exhausted. He had endured two weeks straight of debilitating treatment.

We had pushed Linda Granger more than we had pushed anyone. But her tumors had not shrunk. Mr. Jensen was stronger than she and seemed capable of tolerating treatment more than she had been able to. And I felt desperate, as desperate as I have ever felt in my life.

I decided that if possible I would push Mr. Jensen even harder than we had pushed her. We would repeat the entire cycle of treatment on him.

We pheresed him again four days in a row. On January 25, his platelet count dropped so low I considered it unsafe to give him a full dose of IL-2, but we did infuse LAK cells mixed with some IL-2. This was repeated on January 27 and 28.

That was his last treatment. His platelet count simply dropped too low to give him anything else.

His weight had risen from 209 pounds to 233 pounds, but after IL-2 was stopped it was quickly returning to normal. His kidney function had become abnormal but that, too, was recovering quickly. On January 29, as soon as it was clear he was no longer in any danger and the changes in his lungs due to the excess fluid had cleared, we sent him downstairs for a routine chest X ray.

Nothing about it was routine. The X ray marked a dividing line in my life, and my memory of it remains vivid.

I was sitting at my desk with the doors to my office closed. Usually I keep them open, an invitation to people to walk in. The fact that they were closed warned everyone that I was working and to interrupt me only for something important.

There was a knock on the door and it opened. Steve Ettinghausen pushed his head in somewhat hesitantly. I glanced up.

"Dr. Rosenberg," he said, "I think you'll be interested in seeing this X ray."

I told him to come in. Everything in my office—bookshelves, desk, a small conference table, computer—seems crammed together, almost as if shoved into the middle of the room. There is a small X-ray viewing screen squeezed between a blackboard and the door.

Steve slapped two X rays onto the screen and switched on the high-intensity light. I came over from my desk.

On the left he put up Mr. Jensen's pretreatment lung X ray. It showed one very large lesion and numerous small ones. On the right was the new X ray. I stared at it.

The large tumor had shrunk. There was no question of the shrinkage. The smaller ones had disappeared. There was no sign of the smaller ones at all.

It was as if someone had kicked me in the stomach.

My God! I thought. *All the years I have waited for a result like this. Can it be real? Can it have finally happened?*

I stood for a moment, silent, thinking of everything—everything!—that had gone before, staring at the X rays, fixing their images in my mind, my eyes darting from the left to the right and back again. *Is it possible? Is this really happening?*

The X rays were real and as their reality sank in, I was suffused with a combination of excitement—wanting to shout out loud and allow myself to erupt—and fear, fear that the X ray was misleading.

"We've got to do immediate lung tomograms," I said.

A tomogram is also an X ray but a much more definitive and quantitative one; tomograms focus at different, precise depths of the lung and can show different slices of tissue. It was possible, just possible, that Jensen's tumors remained unchanged, and that the chest X ray had simply failed to pick them up for some reason. But they would appear in tomograms. We tried to schedule Jensen for tomograms. It was too late. We could not get them done that day.

Despite my concerns, I was excited enough to call Alice and my brother. I told them, "I think we may have seen tumor shrinkage in a patient but the key will be tomorrow's X rays."

That night at dinner I could barely contain myself. My children picked up on my excitement and grew excited, too. I told them nothing was certain until the next day's X rays. In the morning Alice gave them an extra quarter to call me from school to find out the results. They did.

Steve Ettinghausen kept calling downstairs to find out when the X rays were ready. The instant they were, he picked me up in my office. Together we walked down the stairs, winding around corridors, past patients waiting for tests, down to the X ray reading area. I felt as though I was holding my breath the entire way down. Steve brought out an earlier tomogram for comparison. We put the new one side by side with the old one.

The large tumor had shrunk by more than half. The smaller ones had in fact disappeared. There was no question of this. We could clearly see what the official X ray report later concluded: "There is strong suggestive evidence of diminution of size of all the metastatic deposits demonstrated, with the disappearance of several."

I turned to Steve, clenched my fist, and said, *"Yes!"*

From there we went straight to see Mr. Jensen. His wife was in the room when we told him.

"It looks like your tumors are shrinking," I said excitedly.

He was pleased but calm and almost matter-of-fact. He replied, "Yeah, I knew this was going to work."

His comment and manner stunned me for a moment. It reminded me of all the other patients I had treated. They had all expected their treatments to work, too. The memory of them and of their trust in me made me, for a moment, turn inward.

A response in one isolated patient meant little. Mr. DeAngelo had cured himself. I would not allow myself to grow too excited.

Fifteen days later, on February 13, 1985, Linda Granger returned to the clinic for her follow-up appointment. There is a waiting area by several large windows, a nurse's station, a conference room for the doctors, fellows, and nurses, and a dozen examination rooms. She was waiting for me in the second room on the left, just past the nurses' station. I walked in and barely got the opportunity to ask, "How are you feeling?"

"My tumors are going away!" she declared.

Immediately we measured them. *She was right!* Quickly we did another biopsy. The pathologist concluded the specimen was "probably totally necrotic."

Her tumors were dead. They were dead. And now they were disappearing.

Jensen had thrilled me but measuring Linda Granger's tumors and later seeing the pathology report gave me confidence that what we had seen was real.

Linda Granger returned again for a complete series of tests on March 20. I was tense awaiting the results. It is not uncommon for radiation and chemotherapy to cause short-lived shrinkage of some tumors, after which the tumor starts growing again. Perhaps we had achieved only a similarly temporary result.

Her tumors had all been palpable to the touch. Now there was no sign of cancer found by either physical evaluation or any other test. She was a complete response.

Her cancer had disappeared.

When Linda Granger entered our protocol she was expected to live no more than a few months. The three-year survival rate of her illness was zero. The Navy had discharged her. Instead, three years later she was petitioning the Navy for return to active duty. The Navy had no idea how to respond to her condition. The Bethesda Naval Hospital stated that people in her situation died and she should not be returned to active duty. Her father urged her to fight, arguing that if she returned to active duty people would no longer see her as "the dying cancer patient."

"He was right," she says. "It was my first opening back into the real world, where there weren't sick people, where I wasn't surrounded by sick people and tests."

Returning to the Navy required the intervention of the Secretary of the Navy, who overrode a disability review board and also promoted her to commander—so she kept pace with her class and to ensure that her illness would not be held against her. She made it back into the real world after all.

As I write this, more than seven years after her treatment, she continues to have no sign of cancer. She is now executive officer of one of the largest naval bases in the world and still returns for follow-up evaluations every six months.

In the past, when follow-ups were much more frequent, she says, "I always expected bad news. I'd prepare to be brave. When it was good news, I'd party. At the same time I was very afraid. I did not want to set myself up again for disappointment. If anyone ever said I was cured, I'd go ballistic."

But even now there is tension when she returns for her follow-ups. I feel it when I view her X rays. There are no guarantees.

In two patients we had seen tumors shrink, and in one case disappear, after our immunotherapy. After all the deaths, after all the years in the lab, we had found something that worked. For the first time I believed—rather than hoped—that immunotherapy not only could work, but would work. I believed we had taken the first step toward developing a new modality for treating cancer, a modality with enormous potential.

It was a moment of vindication for me, yet it went deeper than vindication. Vindication, like triumph, represents something external, a reaction to the world and to what the world thinks. This was instead one of those rare moments when one feels . . . *satisfied*. Not triumphant or vindicated. Satisfied. Satisfaction speaks to something deep inside oneself, a fulfillment, a peacefulness and fulfillment deeper than triumph can reach.

CHAPTER SEVENTEEN

We quickly began treating as many patients as we could, but this was still only four a week. From these four we were trying to learn both clinical science—how best to administer the treatment—and hard science. And I began to break existing rules about patient care.

When chemotherapy or radiation therapy damages the body, the damage can be irreversible. For this reason we had initially been very cautious in administering IL-2. But in all our patients who received it, the side effects we observed—the weight gain from fluid retention, nausea, fever and chills, kidney and liver dysfunction, low blood counts—disappeared when IL-2 treatment stopped.

We pushed Linda Granger to the edge of death, but even in her case her kidney, liver, and other functions returned quickly to normal. We pushed James Jensen until his platelet count fell to a life-threatening level, and his platelet count quickly rebounded. Follow-up appointments confirmed that neither patient had suffered any lingering damage.

Because of this I thought we might be able to push harder and further with IL-2 than one can with chemotherapeutic agents. Since higher dosages of IL-2 seemed to have greater impact on cancer, I decided to see just how hard we could in fact push.

Siona Willoughby was a fifty-four-year-old single woman, short and overweight and the mother of grown children. She was suffering from widely metastatic kidney cancer.

I decided to begin her treatment in the ICU, push harder than we had ever pushed, and monitor her very closely. If her blood pressure dropped, we would treat it but continue the IL-2. If her platelet count dropped, we would give her platelets but continue the IL-2. If her breathing became labored, we would put her on oxygen but continue the IL-2.

In addition to the routine monitoring devices on all ICU patients, including an EKG, we put in a Swan-Ganz catheter, which measures pressure on both sides of the heart, and an arterial cannula in the radial artery in her wrist, which measures blood pressure beat by beat. A nurse was in constant attendance, no more than a few feet away.

I began her treatment with 720,000 units of IL-2 per kilogram of body weight—ten times what Mr. Jensen started with—by bolus injection three times a day, and pheresed her according to the procedure we used for Mr. Jensen. And we pushed. We pushed hard enough that even some of the nurses in the ICU were uncomfortable with what I was doing.

We examined blood tests three times a day, watched every monitor, and we pushed ahead, giving her more IL-2. She did develop serious side effects, and her blood pressure dropped to a dangerous level. Normally low blood pressure is alleviated by adding volume—giving blood, plasma, or other solutions—but adding volume would only exacerbate fluid loss into her lungs. So we tried a different technique, administering vasopressors early in the course of treatment. These drugs cause small blood vessels to contract, squeezing the blood supply into a smaller space and thus increasing blood pressure. They worked. Her blood pressure rose. And we continued to give her IL-2.

After treatment ended, she recovered from the side effects rapidly.

She also responded to the therapy. We watched most of her tumors melt away. The next two patients with kidney cancer also responded. Their tumors shrank dramatically.

We were rewriting the rules.

Treatment became standardized. We gave two cycles: The first lasted four to five days, followed by five days of pheresis, followed in turn by a second four to five days of infusions. Later we treated most patients on the ward, transferring to the ICU only those who required close monitoring.

Patients knew that others had responded. They talked to each other during treatment. Their families talked to each other's families. We tried to be guarded and conservative, but patients sensed our own optimism. Hope surged through the ward.

Yet the treatment still did not help most patients. Rounds became emotionally charged. We would walk into one room where a patient was responding—sometimes we could see the tumor shrinking from one day to the next—and we were all euphoric. After all the years of failure, each success was a special thrill. But in the next room, or the next bed, would be a patient who was not responding. Each failure was more difficult to bear.

Clinic was similarly charged. I spent all Tuesday and Thursday afternoons there, assessing the results of treatment in old patients and evaluating potential new ones. These were tense times; the routine and the tension remain similar today.

Follow-up assessments began six weeks after treatment and continued indefinitely for those patients who responded or whom we continued to treat. Don White, a computer specialist who had joined our group, generated a list each week of the status of all the patients we had treated and were following. Most patients underwent X rays, CAT scans, MRIs, and other tests the day preceding their clinic appointment. The next morning the research nurses, clinical fellows, and I gathered in a room with walls of viewing screens. We filled the screens with scans and searched shadows for shadows, analyzed the most subtle of chiaroscuros. To those who are not doctors, our terms must seem odd, so precise and almost oxymoronic. Like the reversal of darkness and light on X rays, good words become bad and bad words become good. *A lymph node is negative.* There is no sign of cancer, which improves the chances of containing the disease. *A patient progresses.* But the progress referred to is of the tumor; the patient's cancer has grown.

When we saw evidence of tumor growth, we silently removed

the signs of failure and slipped the films back into the files. A sense of sadness and personal failure permeated the room. I had to remind myself that we had not caused the cancer and we were doing our best. Yet I wondered if we were; if we worked harder, might we do better? And I began to prepare myself; a few hours later I would have to tell this patient that the treatment had not worked.

But the scans that showed tumor shrinkage—these were a joy. We left these scans up on our viewbox and admired them, stopped colleagues walking by and insisted that they admire them, too.

These moments examining scans were as tense as I have ever experienced. For the patients, the tension waiting for word from us must have been as close to unbearable as anything can be.

Seeing patients in follow-up could be difficult. The clinic waiting area was furnished like that at an airport gate, the chairs cushioned but not quite comfortable. There could be no comfort in waiting, waiting to be summoned to a private room. The clinic was generally silent. Most patients came with a parent or a spouse, and some older patients came with children. Yet the patients were alone. One either has cancer or one does not; it is not an experience to be shared. Even between the closest people there is separation in this, a separation sensed by both parties. Patients, waiting, stayed within themselves. During treatment, patients on the wards often became friendly with one another, but only rarely here.

There was no single emotion present, only intensity. Often, under the pressure of the disease and the situation, superficialities and constraints were stripped away. Some people discovered reserves of strength they had not known they had. Most people became more of what they were: Optimists became more optimistic; pessimists became more pessimistic; giving people became more giving; irritable people became more difficult. One woman whose cancer disappeared entirely—and has not recurred—told me that she got angry several weeks before each scheduled follow-up, angry at everyone and everything. A few patients were jealous. Linda Granger became friendly with one who was dying. She recalled one follow-up visit: "I felt guilty I did so well. Her family did not react well to me."

These patients had one thing in common: We were their last hope. Doctors had previously told virtually all our patients that they had no hope. In *Paradise Lost* Milton wrote, "So farewell hope, and with hope farewell fear."

Without hope, and even without fear, one loses one's humanity. Nothing matters, including life. Many patients have told me that their worst experience was having hope taken from them, and that we had given them hope again. Even if our treatments failed, as terrible as that was, most patients were appreciative. Their participation in an experimental therapy gave them purpose and a sense of contributing again.

I knew how anxious these patients were. When I sat down with them in an examining room I did not keep them in suspense. If the treatment had worked, my first words were, "The news is good."

If the news was not good, I first asked patients how they were feeling, if all side effects had dissipated, but then I was straightforward. "It looks like your tumors are growing," I would say and immediately discuss alternative treatment plans that we could consider. Even though nothing would be effective long-term, we could usually offer some short-term solution to a symptom. And even if we could not do that, I wanted my patients to know we would not abandon them.

It became an almost unbearable roller coaster for me. The thrill I got from seeing a cancer shrink, and from giving a patient this news, has never gone away, nor has the pain of walking into one of those small rooms and telling a patient who has already failed every alternative that our treatment, too, has failed. Before we had ever seen a response, failure had been difficult to accept. But we had been attempting something that no one had ever achieved. Now that we had seen successes, each patient who did not respond became our failure and our responsibility in a new and deeper way.

Some who did not respond were apologetic, as if they had let us down. Many thanked me gratefully even when the treatment failed. This was particularly difficult for me.

The patients could not understand why the treatment worked for some but not for others. Neither did I. When I told them this, they seemed to feel better, reassured that they were not responsible for the failure. One man, told that the treatment had not worked, urged me not to get discouraged. How could I answer him?

I pushed harder.

The term "objective response" in cancer research refers to a specific measure of success in treating patients. A complete response is defined by the disappearance of all signs of cancer in a patient for at least one month. A partial response is defined by shrinkage of the total tumor burden by at least 50 percent, no appearance of new tumors, and no growth of any existing tumor; this shrinkage and lack of growth must also remain for at least one month.

All patients whom we treated had failed to respond to any other therapy and had no other effective treatments available to them. Linda Granger experienced a complete response. James Jensen experienced a partial response. Siona Willoughby experienced a partial response. When we had treated twelve patients and five had experienced objective responses, we submitted an article about the therapy to *The New England Journal of Medicine*.

The journal editors understood the significance of the report and asked me to modify the article to include more patients. After treating twenty-five patients, eleven of whom experienced objective responses, we resubmitted the article.

The *New England Journal* article would attract enormous attention. Yet before its appearance, I would already have training in the public aspects of medicine.

. . .

On Friday evening, July 12, 1985, on my way home from work I listened to the radio and heard that President Ronald Reagan had just arrived at Bethesda Naval Hospital. Not long after I got home, Captain Dale Oller, whom I did not know, called, identified himself as chief of general surgery at the naval hospital, and asked, "Would you be willing to help us on a special case?"

"Is it the president?"

"Yes. But I prefer not to talk on the phone. Can you come over?"

By the time I arrived, hordes of reporters already occupied the parking lot, along with the trailers of equipment and technicians for network television, ropes to contain them all, and Secret Service. I made my way through the crowd into the hospital to Oller's office, where he and several other physicians were conferring.

The meeting made me aware of a flaw in medical treatment provided to the president. Except for emergency situations, such as the assassination attempt on Reagan in 1981, if hospitalized, the president always goes to the Bethesda Naval Hospital. But the president is treated by whoever happens to be on rotation. If the finest doctor in the Navy happens to be on rotation, then the president is lucky. But the least capable doctor in the Navy could just as easily treat the president.

In this case, the president received excellent care. Dale Oller is an experienced and competent surgeon. But he was not a cancer specialist and was not required—other than his obligation to the patient—to seek help when he ventured outside his own area of expertise.

My conversation with Oller and the other physicians was extended and detailed. Everything I learned was later revealed to the press. Fourteen months earlier Reagan had been advised to have a colonoscopy but had put it off. Only recently had he agreed to the procedure. The colonoscopy had revealed a growth. Other tests to determine the likelihood of metastatic deposits had already been performed and were negative. The results were before me.

Oller wanted a judgment from me as to whether an operation the next day was reasonable. I agreed that it made sense. Oller, who would perform it, asked me to participate in case of unforeseen complications. Although preoperative tests had shown no evidence of metastatic cancer, it would not be unusual to find potentially dangerous metastases that scans had not revealed.

I went home that night and returned to the hospital at 7:00 A.M. and, with Oller, met Reagan for the first time. I was impressed by his manner. He was one of those rare patients who always try to make the doctors feel better, and he had an Irish charm and a sense of social ease, which I saw in Alice. He signed a document transferring presidential authority to George Bush, was anesthetized, and the operation began.

Oller did a flawless job resecting approximately two feet of the colon. Experience with prominent patients had taught me that it is a mistake to change a routine for them; unpredictable and dangerous things can result. So we decided not to allow Secret Service personnel in the O.R. They were intimidating enough standing outside the door with automatic weapons drawn, confiscating every bandage and needle that touched the president— explaining that they wanted no souvenirs to be collected.

The lesion itself, a villous adenoma, looked very suspicious. I thought it was cancerous, although we would not know for certain until the pathologists finished analyzing it forty-eight hours later, on Monday. We examined the abdomen and saw no indication of any metastases.

The operation took two hours and fifty-three minutes. Immediately afterward, and after speaking with Nancy Reagan, the entire surgical team, still dressed in greens, met the press in a large auditorium.

It was an almost surreal experience at first. As we walked in, the first thing that struck me was a blinding blaze of spotlights, followed immediately by an incredible and deafening roar as hundreds of cameras clicked and their automatic mechanisms wound film to frame after frame. The first four rows of the auditorium were filled with photographers, and the roar of their cameras fell off slowly but never stopped. Most questions about cancer were referred or directed to me.

That night I began to learn more about the press. Print and

broadcast reporters called, probably a hundred or more, each one insistent. I talked with none of them. No effort had been made by anyone in the White House to have any of the physicians do anything except present all the facts openly. The president himself had wanted us to speak openly at the press conference, and I had already done so; all relevant information was already out. Beyond that I would not comment and even what I write here was all revealed at the press conferences. The president had the same rights to a confidential doctor-patient relationship as anyone else.

Sunday I went to the lab. Between the operation and the press conference Saturday, I had missed only nine hours of work, but it seemed as if I had been gone for weeks. It was good to get back—for a day. That evening Alice and I continued our Sunday routine; we saw a movie, a western called *Silverado*.

White House Chief of Staff Donald Regan and spokesman Larry Speakes had asked me to attend the press conference to be held after the pathology report appeared on Monday. It was supposed to begin at 10:00 A.M., but we waited four hours for the pathologists to finish. Evidently they rewrote their report many times to make it perfect. Finally we got it. Regan and Speakes watched while Oller and I read it carefully. It was not good news. The president had a cancer with some invasion of the colon. Still, in well over 50 percent of cases the operation he had undergone would be completely curative. No additional therapy was required.

At Regan's request, I spoke with Nancy Reagan before seeing the president. I often see a spouse first; it gives the spouse a chance to adjust and prepare to support the patient—rather than break down at bad news. She reacted as any concerned wife would, emotionally, but quickly regained her self-control. We then went to see the president.

He occupied a suite that seemed designed more for him to run the government than relax, with anterooms and very likely all the communications equipment necessary for the White House to function. His own room was very comfortable, very well furnished, and very large; his standard hospital bed seemed strangely out of place in it. Briefly I explained the diagnosis and its implications. He listened, took the news well, and returned to his book.

From there, Speakes, Oller, and I immediately wound our way down a maze of back stairs and corridors into the auditorium for the press conference. The reporters had been waiting for hours.

The press conference seemed oddly familiar to me. I felt as if I was about to talk to a concerned family, and that my role was to give them all the facts but also be reassuring. The facts were far from terrible; the likelihood that the operation had cured the patient was more than 50 percent. As I looked out at the crowd, I saw concern on the faces of these people. It reflected that of the country beyond, but it was also the same concern I saw on a daily basis in the families of my patients.

Oller began by basically reading the pathologist's conclusions. I had expected to stand at his side and answer only specific questions about cancer, as had happened two days earlier. But Oller finished his technical recitation, announced that I would make some comments, and moved away from the microphone. It took a moment to focus, and I sensed confusion among the reporters as to the precise nature and circumstances of the president's disease. Oller had used the word "adenocarcinoma," but he had buried it among other technical terms. It seemed that not all the reporters had heard it or understood its significance. In addition, his very reluctance to use the word "cancer" reflected part of what makes the disease so frightening. Cancer patients feel isolated because no one wants to use the word around them. There is a need to demystify both the disease and the word, make it less frightening and isolating, and only using the word will do that.

I stepped up to the microphone and said, "The president has cancer."

Unwittingly I had just spoken what would become a headline in practically every major paper in the world the next day. I then proceeded to explain the precise nature of the president's disease. The reporters asked many of the same questions family members ask, and I had answered these same questions many times in the small anterooms outside our surgical suites.

I received many calls from the press for the next few weeks, but did not comment further. The president's convalescence proceeded smoothly. I immediately returned to work.

CHAPTER EIGHTEEN

*T*he *New England Journal of Medicine* occupies a unique place among scientific journals. Its articles deal only with important clinical findings, and its imprimatur increases the visibility of these findings. Studies that first appear in it are routinely reported by major papers in the country and on network newscasts.

Editors at *The New England Journal* distribute advance copies of the publication to journalists under an embargo; in exchange for getting advance copies, journalists agree not to report on findings prior to their publication in *The New England Journal*. The journal's editors justify this practice by arguing that it gives reporters time to research stories and place new findings in context. But it also can lead to sensationalism by allowing, if not encouraging, journalists to build up their stories. I think the disadvantages outweigh the advantages.

It was clear our findings would attract attention. We had treated twenty-five cancer patients who had failed other therapies and were considered terminal; eleven of them had responded.

Arnold Relman, then the editor of the journal, recognized the potential impact of these results. In an effort to dampen the media reaction to the article and inject a note of caution, he asked me to change the title from "Treatment with" LAK and IL-2 to "Observations on" this therapy. I did, but this subtle change had no effect.

But between the time the article was accepted and its publication, a clinical tragedy occurred.

Gary Fowlke was the thirty-fifth patient in the LAK-plus-IL-2 protocol. He suffered from melanoma that had spread throughout his lungs and liver. A twenty-four-year-old mechanic from Illinois, burly, enthusiastic, vital, and built like a defensive tackle, he practically bounded into the clinic. He flirted with the nurses and strolled up and down the ward telling jokes and keeping the spirits of fellow patients up. The contrast between his outward appearance of health and vitality and the inward state of his body, the mortal danger into which his cancer had put him, was as great as in any patient I have ever seen.

He was referred to us in early August 1985, and we performed a wide excision and removed all the lymph nodes in his left axilla. Nine of twenty-one lymph nodes were positive, a terrible sign. Within weeks after surgery, new metastatic lesions appeared on his back, X rays revealed tumors in both lungs, and his lymph nodes were swollen. He seemed in excellent health yet had a virulent, extremely aggressive cancer.

We offered him the combined LAK-IL-2 therapy. He accepted. There was so much hope in him. He kept a diary and filled it with his determination to beat his disease, to see a friend's baby, to find a woman to spend the rest of his life with.

Mr. Fowlke received a series of high doses of IL-2, beginning September 18, 1985, and continuing for several days. Then we stopped. On Monday, September 23, we pheresed him and did so for five days straight. That Friday the IL-2 doses recommenced, and he also received two LAK infusions. These infusions of both LAK and IL-2 continued until October 1.

Then his blood pressure dropped into the eighties and we administered dopamine, one of the vasopressors we used. His kidney function dropped below 10 percent of normal, and he became restless, then agitated, occasionally tugging at the IV lines, and confused. We stopped further treatment.

Still, he recovered very quickly—so quickly we sent him home the day after his treatment ended. All his tests returned to normal. So on Monday, October 7, we brought him back for a second cycle of treatment, again pheresed him five days in a row and restarted his IL-2. We treated him in the ICU, where we could monitor him closely.

Treatment continued uninterrupted until October 11. Again his blood pressure fell and kidney function became abnormal. We halted his IL-2 and treated his symptoms, as we had done with other patients and earlier with him.

His symptoms abated, and we resumed giving him IL-2—although only one dose on Sunday and Monday, October 13 and 14. That Monday he also received two LAK infusions.

Mr. Fowlke began to get agitated again and seemed to be having trouble. On Tuesday, October 15, we gave him one more dose of IL-2. He grew more agitated. We decided to cease treatment and called in our psychiatric consult. His oxygenation was low—his pO2 was 53—so he was given oxygen, which quickly raised his pO2 to normal, 123. The psychiatrist prescribed Haldol, a powerful sedative, and he calmed down initially, but throughout the day his agitation and disorientation gradually increased.

On October 16, his blood gases were good but his creatinine, which measures kidney function, remained high. A chest X ray showed much fluid in the lungs. His white blood cell count was mildly elevated. Normally, elevated white counts are indicators of infection, but IL-2 distorts those counts. A nurse who sat constantly by his bedside noted at 4:00 P.M. that he was restless and disoriented.

Abruptly, at 5:15 P.M., his heart rate dropped from 140 to 115, held there only briefly, then dropped further—to 88 with irregular beats. His respiration became shallow and he became cyanotic. The nurse called a Code Blue.

Then his heart stopped.

I heard the Code Blue call over the loudspeaker and rushed down the hall. By the time I arrived the team was working to resuscitate him. He had already been intubated and external cardiac compression was being administered, which keeps blood circulating even if the heart has stopped.

We shocked his heart. It began to beat again, weakly, but stopped.

We shocked it again. It beat weakly, then stopped again.

We injected adrenaline directly into the heart muscle. It had no effect.

Nothing we did was working. We continued to administer cardiac compression. His heart would not start. I could not understand why we could not make progress. People die on the street from cardiac arrest, but in an ICU with a nurse watching, with state-of-the-art technology and drugs and expert care available instantly, it is often possible to resuscitate them.

But we could not make progress.

We had been working on him for more than an hour. I decided to open his chest and directly massage his heart. This was a technique that had largely been replaced by external cardiac compression. But external compression had not succeeded. Quickly I made a long incision in the fourth interspace, put in a rib-spreader, felt for his heart, found it, and began to massage it. I massaged his heart for twenty more minutes as we continued to administer volume and drugs.

We could not start Gary Fowlke's heart beating.

We had begun trying to resuscitate him at 5:15 P.M. We tried everything we knew, everything that was standard procedure, everything that was extraordinary. Nothing worked. At 7:00 P.M. we declared Gary Fowlke dead.

The autopsy revealed cancer throughout his body. He had more than twenty tumors in his liver. He had multiple cancer deposits in all the lobes of the lung. As healthy as he had seemed, he could not have survived more than another few months.

But cancer had not killed him. In fact, the pathology report noted that the tumors had some necrosis and were infiltrated by lymphocytes.

His lungs were in a state of acute distress caused in part by a massive infection. Gram-positive bacteria were found in his muscle tissue, brain, and lungs. His liver was also congested. The pathologist could not locate the original source of the infection.

The treatment had killed him.

IL-2 had hindered his ability to fight the infection. IL-2 had also caused him to retain fluid, which partially filled his lungs and helped create his respiratory distress.

There had been no warning of his condition, at least none that we could recognize. He had developed fevers but they were consistent with common side effects of IL-2, so we had not suspected an infection. His white count, while slightly elevated, had also not given us enough information to suspect the infection.

It was the first time in my life that my attempt to help a patient had instead killed him. It was a debilitating, numbing feeling. He had bounded into the Surgery Branch and filled it with his vitality. Now he was dead.

Intellectually I knew treatment-related deaths were inevitable, particularly when we were first learning how to treat people. Linda Granger had come far too close to dying, and I understood there was an enormous amount we did not know about IL-2's side effects. Intellectually, I knew that we were treating terminal patients in desperate situations. Intellectually, I sought solace in the fact that treatment-related deaths in other regimens were considerably higher than we had yet seen.

Still . . .

Gary Fowlke's death rippled through all of us. It shocked all of us. In an operation, a doctor may do everything right but complications that are impossible to foresee may arise, and the patient dies. At least the doctor knows he or she did everything possible, everything according to the guidelines. Here there were no guidelines. That made all of us question our judgment, wonder what, if we had done it differently, would have saved Gary Fowlke.

I still do not know the answer to that. But the experience emphasized to us that IL-2 masked white counts. This made us all more aware of the danger of infection and helped later patients. I also began to use antibiotics much more aggressively than most doctors are taught to do.

At the same time, I was concerned that the tragedy would intimidate some of the people on the clinical team, make them—or myself—pull back and treat our other patients less aggressively. Some people in the hospital had been saying that we pushed too hard. The nurses in our ICU and on our 2 East Ward, whose commitment to patients equaled our own, were shocked by the death. Some of them wanted to stop treatment to other patients when I wanted to push ahead. It was my decision so we did continue, but tensions arose. I did not want that. The nurses' trust in the treatment course mattered to me and to the patients. I had no choice but to continue to push.

I tried to keep everyone's spirits up. It was impossible. Rounds became quiet, very quiet.

Mr. Fowlke's mother wrote letters to me and told me about him, what he was like, that he knew his situation was serious but that he had confidence in us. It was as if she was trying simultaneously to absolve me of blame and make certain that I knew him. She wanted to make him a whole person to me. It reminded me once again of the Holocaust. Those who suffered in it had most feared not being remembered.

It was a dark time.

Gary Fowlke's death occurred after *The New England Journal* had accepted our article but before publication. By the time the article appeared, we had treated more than 100 men and women, including all our immunotherapy patients in our earlier Phase I studies. We pushed hard, but we were pushing terminally ill patients for whom no alternative therapy could work, and who knew of the risks and consented to them.

Of the first twenty-five LAK and IL-2 patients reported in the *New England Journal* study, two—Linda Granger and one other patient—had to be intubated. Twenty suffered some shortness of breath. Sixteen retained enough fluid to gain more than 10 percent of their body weight. Infections at the site of the central intravenous line occurred at an increased rate. (A later randomized protocol studying this problem showed we could control it by administering prophylactic doses of antibiotics, but in the early stages of the treatment—when we were only just realizing that treatment increased the risk of infection—we did not do this.)

I understood that significant dangers remained, and that only experience could teach us about them. We all understood this, including the patients. Still, considering the fact that we were attempting to develop an entirely new mode of therapy, I considered our safety record to be as good as possible.

And as we began to learn what danger signs to look for, as we confirmed that all side effects were reversible—and now that we knew our therapy could cause tumors to regress and even disappear—we became, if anything, even more aggressive.

While we were learning these things, while the tragedy of Gary Fowlke still hung over both the lab and the clinic, in late November 1985, ten days before *The New England Journal* was scheduled to publish our article, *Fortune* ran a cover story. The headline: CANCER BREAKTHROUGH.

The cover photograph was of a vial of liquid, captioned "Cetus Corp.'s tumor-zapping interleukin-2." The story began: "Cautious cancer researchers fear the familiar phrase 'cancer breakthrough' almost as much as they dread the word cancer itself. But these days even the most careful researchers are having trouble containing their excitement about a striking family of biological compounds as a way to treat cancer. So powerful are the new weapons that many clinicians believe the odds in the struggle against cancer will soon be tipped in favor of the patient."

The opening sentence was correct. "Cancer breakthrough" is exactly the hyperbole scientists want to avoid.

I had refused to be interviewed for the article or cooperate in any way, and the reporter mentioned my refusal. But he did not need my cooperation or my comments. He had much of my data anyway. There were only three possible sources: someone in my lab, which I doubted very much; someone at *The New England Journal of Medicine*, which I also doubted strongly; and Cetus, which had much to gain from the story. Incensed, I called both chief executive officer Robert Fildes and president Jeff Price at Cetus. Both swore no one there had leaked the information.

Dozens of calls came in after the *Fortune* story. I explained that I could not make any comment until after the *New England*

Journal article appeared. One call came from Tom Brokaw, who asked to come on rounds with me and promised to honor the *New England Journal* embargo. I agreed. I also agreed to other embargoed interviews with several other reporters. When the advance issues of the journal were delivered to many more journalists, even more interview requests poured in.

Every reporter also wanted to speak with a patient. I debated whether to allow it or not. At the time, we were treating a patient who had melanoma; his tumors were literally melting away between cycles of treatment. We were pheresing him that week and when I mentioned the media requests to him, he was eager to appear on television.

I told several journalists, including Brokaw, that they could interview him as long as I was present to correct any factual misstatements he might make about the therapy. I now believe that allowing the interview was an error of judgment on my part. I should have foreseen that it would exaggerate the benefits of the therapy and further sensationalize the story. I should have refused to make patients available, and have never allowed an in-hospital patient interview since.

More than a year after we treated Linda Granger, in the Thursday, December 5, 1985, issue, listed as a "special report," *The New England Journal of Medicine* published the findings. Despite the dozens of calls I had received over the preceding weeks and the several embargoed interviews I had given, the reaction astonished me.

Both NBC and ABC led their evening newscasts with a report on the article. CBS also ran the story but not as its lead.

The New York Times, the *Los Angeles Times, USA Today, The Washington Post*, the *Chicago Tribune*, and others put the story on the front page the next day. Papers around the world—in Italy, France, China, Japan, Great Britain—ran the story on the front page. *Time* ran a major, lengthy piece on it. And *Newsweek* put me on its cover.

Perhaps because of my involvement with Ronald Reagan, perhaps because of the *Fortune* story, which had sensitized journalists to the findings, the report suddenly became a major news event.

I was not so naive as to have expected the report of my findings to pass without notice. But I had expected nothing like this.

Even before the network news shows, as radio newscasts announced the findings during the day, the phone calls began. After the network newscasts they continued through the night. The next day, after the headlines in the morning papers, literally thousands of telephone calls overwhelmed the NCI and NIH switchboards. A contract screening service soon began taking our calls. Other cancer centers around the country were similarly inundated. Alexander Fefer at the University of Washington's Fred Hutchinson Cancer Center told *The Boston Globe*, "Oh my God, it started when I was awakened this morning and it hasn't stopped yet." He added, "Deep down I am concerned about the amount of publicity it has gotten."

I was concerned, too. The reaction was disturbing, even frightening. The words "cancer breakthrough" were seen in many headlines, though I tried to be cautious in my comments and never used the phrase. I was treating four patients a week. Hundreds of people a day were calling, seeking treatment. I had never seen anything like this, nor known of it.

Reading descriptions of what my lab was doing in the lay press was a new experience for me and a disorienting one. The recognition of the work's importance excited me and I was proud of what we had accomplished, but I knew its limitations. So did every other scientist. Not all patients responded. Far from it. Not all those who did respond continued to do so. Although Linda Granger continues free of cancer today, seven years after her treatment, Mr. Jensen's cancer recurred and killed him. We had not cured cancer. We had only detected a crack in its stone face.

The NCI press office asked me to hold a press conference. I refused. A press conference, which to me resembles hawking one's wares, seemed inappropriate. I also feared that in a press conference I lacked control. I could never control a story a reporter wrote, but in a one-on-one interview I could at least evaluate whether or not a reporter understood me. The reporter's questions would tell me that; if the reporter did not understand something, I could correct it. In a press conference, distortions and inaccuracies could arise inadvertently or from sloppiness. So I talked to reporters in individual interviews.

In those interviews, with an increasing sense of urgency I tried to play down the expectations. Stories did begin to sound more constrained. That weekend Vince DeVita and I were invited to appear on "Face the Nation" on CBS. We agreed.

Vince arrived in the studio first that Sunday morning and mentioned the tragedy of Gary Fowlke. While we waited to go on and sat talking casually, Leslie Stahl, the host of the show, came back to say hello. She said that she understood there had been a death. Her comment was made casually, but I could sense much more than casual interest.

It suddenly became clear to me how she must see the situation. As often as I had thought of Gary Fowlke in the preceding few weeks, I had never before thought of making public his death until now.

The very concept of offering the press a running scorecard on patients—who responded, who did not respond, who died—offended me. The place to publish scientific information is in a scientific journal. Had the death occurred in one of the twenty-five patients included in the *New England Journal* study, it would have been reported. It would be reported, along with any other treatment-related deaths, in our next scientific article.

Another reason for not revealing the death was that I did not consider it unexpected. To the contrary, some deaths were inevitable.

But as this issue evolved, I came to realize that most people, including journalists, do not realize how much danger cancer treatments, and especially experimental cancer treatments, can carry. For example, a *New England Journal of Medicine* study reporting on an experimental therapy involving bone marrow transplants and aggressive chemotherapy revealed twenty-one treatment-related deaths out of 100 patients. In an experimental regimen combining radiation and chemotherapy for lung cancer at the University of Washington, reported in *The Journal of Clinical Oncology*, twelve of seventy-three patients suffered treatment-related deaths. Even in established, nonexperimental chemotherapy regimens, mortality rates—deaths caused by treatment—routinely run from 2 to 5 percent.

These mortality rates are high, but the alternative to treatment is 100 percent mortality. Testicular cancer, for example, was invariably fatal until Larry Einhorn developed a chemotherapy regimen that now cures the vast majority of patients. Yet a *New England Journal* study of the treatment—when it was no longer experimental—reported an overall 4.7 percent treatment-caused mortality rate.

Gary Fowlke was our first treatment-related mortality out of 101 patients with advanced cancer in all our immunotherapy trials. Forty of those 101 patients had by then received the LAK and IL-2 therapy. His death was tragic, but I thought our safety record compared well with the mortality rates of most experimental cancer therapies, particularly since we were in the earliest stages of learning how to care for our patients.

I realized, however, that from a journalist's perspective the death was news, and—perhaps more significant—it was news that seemed to be kept secret. Clearly she would ask me about it on the air. I knew immediately that I had to raise it myself.

In response to the first question she asked, I began to talk about the fact that the treatment was far from perfect. We had found no miracle cure. "The side effects can be quite severe," I said. "We have even seen one death due to the treatment itself."

The next morning I was back in the news again. Every story mentioned the fact that I had announced the information, and it somewhat balanced my failure to announce the death earlier. Still, the delay generated suspicion and criticism.

At the time, I did not fully understand the ramifications of my interactions with the media. At the press conference after Reagan's surgery, I gave reporters all relevant information; clearly in this case the public had a right to know. But after the press conference, I had refused to make any further comment. As a result, reporters sought comments from doctors who had no direct knowledge of the case, and confusion developed.

Partly because of that experience, when my article appeared in *The New England Journal of Medicine* I made myself freely available to the media. But the media reaction to the study spun out of control and I could not contain it. There may be a balance scientists can reach in publicly discussing a scientific development or issue—a balance between the public's right to know and scientists' fears that the public's lack of expertise will lead to misunderstanding or unrealistic expectations—but in this case I failed to reach it.

Now immunotherapy was evolving into a "story," with controversy and angles and science politics. In the aftermath of the reporting on the death, I think, some reporters became suspicious of immunotherapy. Their suspicion would later have repercussions.

CHAPTER NINETEEN

Vince DeVita immediately moved to establish Clinical Centers outside NIH to administer immunotherapy. These outside centers would attempt to confirm our findings, expand our knowledge about the treatment, and widen the patient base. Vince also intended to make this happen quickly.

Even before the publication of our *New England Journal* paper, NCI officials began making discreet phone calls to respected clinicians in cancer centers. David Parkinson, a doctor then at Tufts Medical Center in Boston and now with us, received one of the calls and later said, "I was asked, 'If there was an opportunity to give a biological therapy [which meant IL-2], and if NCI paid for it, would you be interested in doing it and how fast could you get a proposal in?' It was clear what was being talked about. I had heard the *New England Journal* paper was coming. I said, 'Are you kidding? Of course.' "

Within a few days after publication, Vince announced that NCI would fund six IL-2 pilot programs in existing cancer centers around the country, and used his authority to shift $2.5 million from other areas for them. Institutions were given only a few weeks to respond. Parkinson said, "The deadline separated the men from the boys. You had to really want this program. I worked all Christmas Day to get the proposal in by the deadline—I think it was December 27."

Despite the tight schedule, more than thirty leading cancer centers competed to be among those chosen. Within a few months after publication of the article, six centers were selected and the heads of each nascent IL-2 program spent a week with us, going on rounds, learning what side effects to expect and how to deal with them, and observing our laboratory techniques. They soon became enthusiastic. While they were here, a patient with metastatic kidney cancer was enjoying a dramatic response; each day on rounds we could see a large tumor on his scapula melt away.

The first reports from the centers confirmed our findings, and they, too, had a good safety record. The six centers combined suffered one treatment death out of their first ninety-four patients. Soon clinicians from around the world were asking to visit the lab or attend our rounds. The requests came often enough that I drafted a form letter in reply to them. The answer was always the same: Yes, come, you are welcome.

Meanwhile we continued to treat four new patients a week. We were driving ourselves to find ways to improve the treatment. We knew only that we had a treatment that worked—sometimes. It was not enough. We needed something more powerful. And in searching for it we discovered an approach that we would eventually use, for the first time in history, to manipulate a patient's genes.

The lab had never stopped working. The moment each of the first responses occurred, word spread rapidly to every investigator, technician, and secretary. Each response sent a jolt of electricity through everyone, and made everyone work harder, made us all focus more intently. The lab meetings every Monday morning, in which two people presented data from their recent experiments, became sharper; the conversations over lunch in the hospital cafeteria heated up; the formal "tea" every Thursday at 4:30 in the amphitheater intensified, the questions became more probing when, after the ritual cookies and coffee and travel slides, one investigator presented his work. Wherever ideas were exchanged—and that meant everywhere, including hallways—people seemed to concentrate harder, think more about what they were saying. At any hour that one walked into the lab, people were working, exploring a dozen paths, hoping that one or more would help us understand the mechanisms of action, and how to improve them.

Earlier, Paul Spiess and I had found that in large enough doses, IL-2 alone caused regression of tumors in mice. Our findings were one reason I had pushed Linda Granger and others so hard. Now Mike Lotze began clinical trials with high-dose IL-2 alone, given every eight hours as we had done in mice. This was far from all we were doing. We studied the impact of a variety of drugs on LAK therapy, searching for synergistic effects. . . . We tried to slow down the elimination of IL-2 from the bloodstream by attaching a large bulky molecule to it. . . . Under a microscope we carefully examined the pattern of tissue destruction by LAK cells, looking for ways to identify, isolate, and grow the most potent cells, the ones that most aggressively attacked cancers. . . . We began experimenting with other interleukins—when we first starting working with IL-2, only two interleukins had been named; there are currently twelve, IL-1 through IL-12. . . . We began studying other proteins, including tumor necrosis factor, or TNF, which can cause tumor destruction by interfering with the blood supply to tumors. . . . We pursued a dozen other leads.

And the most important path we moved down began three weeks before we saw the first response in a patient to LAK and IL-2, on January 11, 1985, when we began a series of experiments that would yield powerful results. It was the six hundredth experiment Paul had performed in his years in my lab and came a relatively short time after we began seeing lymphocytes infiltrating mouse tumors. We began to wonder about this, and to think back.

Our original hypothesis, in 1980, was that the most likely place to find immune cells that recognize and attack cancer cells is within a tumor itself.

That logic had caused me to send Ilana Yron searching inside tumors in the quest for specific killer cells, T lymphocytes uniquely capable of recognizing one animal's cancer and no others. Specific killer cells would, I thought, be the most potent. She had failed to find such specific killing activity. But she had found the nonspecific killing cells we later termed the LAK phenomenon.

We now knew much more about LAK than when Ilana had first encountered them, and we also now knew that lymphocytes, at least some of which were T cells, did infiltrate tumors. We decided to return to the experiments and again study the lymphocytes infiltrating tumors.

Paul performed an experiment in precisely the same way Ilana had five years earlier, except that he used the MCA-105 tumor. Ilana had used the MCA-102 tumor. This seemingly minor, almost coincidental, change turned out to make an enormous difference.

All MCA tumor cell lines were generated the same way: by injecting methylcholanthrene into the same strain of mice. But the cancers that grew were not identical. They developed with subtle differences. It is exactly these subtle differences that make the MCA tumor series a model that closely resembles naturally occurring cancers.

Paul made a single cell suspension from the MCA-105 tumors and grew the lymphocytes from these tumors in IL-2. Exactly as Ilana had seen five years earlier, the lymphocytes grew and killed the cancer cells. In the next two experiments the lymphocytes did not grow. Then on February 6 he grew cells well enough that we decided to compare the therapeutic effects of regular LAK cells with what I later called "tumor-infiltrating lymphocytes," or TIL. So we injected cancer cells into animals and set up several controls.

If TIL cells had the same properties as LAK cells, then animals treated with TIL and LAK should have had approximately the same reduction of cancer. They did not.

Two of the five animals receiving LAK plus IL-2 had no tumors, but one had 151 tumors.

Four animals received TIL and IL-2. Not a single animal had even a single tumor.

The results were too widely scattered to be definitive or statistically significant. But they were suggestive. We had to find out whether the difference was something real and new, something unlike anything Ilana or anyone else had seen, or simply a coincidental distribution of numbers that misleadingly made TIL appear more potent.

Paul immediately tried to repeat the experiment. After several failed attempts to grow lymphocytes, on February 28 he again compared TIL to LAK. But this time the TIL did not kill impressively.

Perhaps the first results meant nothing, and there was no difference between LAK and TIL. But we wanted a definitive answer. We decided to see if we could make the experiment work.

Paul tried again.

On March 15 Paul injected several dozen animals with cancer cells and three days later divided them into five groups. He treated one group with a saline solution for the control; one was treated with IL-2 alone; one with 100 million LAK cells plus IL-2; and two groups with seven to nine million TIL grown from two different MCA-105 tumors. Three days later the animals got a second injection of LAK or TIL.

After two weeks, he sacrificed the animals, extracted their lungs, and began to count lung metastases. We counted up to 250 tumors on each animal's lungs. If there are more than 250 mets on an animal, we write the notation "TNTC," which means "too numerous to count."

One quickly gets headaches from counting. But in this experiment Paul got no headaches. First he became interested, then excited. The mice were coded and he had no idea what treatment these mice had received. Even so, he could tell something special had happened. Many of the mice had no tumors at all. Later he said, "I thought, 'Damn, this is something important. This thing's going to go.'"

All six control animals were TNTC; each had more than 250 tumors.

Four of the five animals treated with IL-2 alone were TNTC, and the fifth had 240 mets.

The five animals receiving LAK plus IL-2 also did not do well in this experiment, probably because there were too few cells given in the second LAK injection to be effective. Two animals were TNTC, one had 244 tumors, one had 216, and one had 163.

Five animals were treated with the TIL grown from one MCA-105, and IL-2. None had a single tumor.

Six animals were treated with the TIL grown from the second MCA-105, and IL-2. None had a single tumor.

Paul and I turned all our energies to examining and extending these results and studying the tumor-infiltrating cells. The experiments consistently showed the remarkable potency of TIL. We began to feel we had found something new and important. Two findings seemed particularly important. One was absolutely critical.

First was TIL's potency. TIL seemed much more powerful than LAK cells. We wanted to find out how much more powerful.

We knew how many LAK cells were needed to effect a cure in our model systems. Paul and I gave fewer and fewer of these new killer cells to see how many of them were required to cure animals. We discovered that as few as one million of the new killer cells had the potency of 100 million LAK cells. The new cells were as much as 100 times more effective than LAK!

On May 1, 1985, at a time when we were vigorously treating patients with LAK and IL-2, we began a more strenuous series of tests of TIL's potency. We had been treating mice with TIL three days after injecting tumor cells, when tumors were still small. Now we waited to treat mice until sixteen days after injecting tumor cells, when tumors had grown bulky and replaced half the animals' lungs. No amount of treatment with LAK cells and IL-2 had ever had any effect in mice with sixteen-day-old tumors.

We also added another element to our treatment. Scientists in other labs had done experiments suggesting that cyclophosphamide, a chemotherapeutic agent, in conjunction with other treatment, helped treat large tumor burdens. We tried cyclophosphamide ourselves.

We judged effectiveness of treatment by observing how long the mice survived, instead of by counting metastases.

At day 50, seven of nine animals in the two groups receiving TIL were still alive. Every animal in every other treatment or control group was dead.

The result thrilled us. Paul was excited: "Cancer is very strong as well as being very clever. People can have pounds of tumor. LAK cells couldn't do anything to that kind of tumor. Now it looked like we might have something that could."

We performed more experiments, refined our methods, extended the experiments to another model involving a different kind of cancer. Paul could barely leave the lab for his excitement, and allowed nothing to interfere. Consistently we got the same results. All animals in all control groups, including those receiving LAK plus IL-2, died. Most animals treated with the combination of TIL, IL-2, and cyclophosphamide lived. This treatment regimen clearly could cure the majority of mice with advanced lung or liver metastases.

TIL were powerful indeed.

But our second finding was even more important.

The results were what we had started out looking for years before. From the first, my approach had been based upon my intuition that tumors have antigens that the immune system can recognize as foreign, and attack.

The lymphocytes growing out of tumors were not LAK cells. We soon conclusively identified them as T lymphocytes, T cells. These T cells could recognize unique antigens on the mouse cancer cells and kill them, and only them. The TIL specifically killed the tumors they grew from; they would not kill other tumors. Their specificity helped explain why they were so much more powerful than LAK cells.

Specific killing by TIL meant that the tumors did have unique antigens. The lock-and-key fit of antigen and receptor was functioning. For the first time in five years, for the first time since we had found the LAK phenomenon, we had returned to the mainstream of immunology.

We realized that five years before, when Ilana Yron had first searched in tumors for T cells that specifically recognized cancers, we had had extraordinarily bad luck. She had been unable to grow these specific cells because she had used MCA-102 tumors, which coincidentally have very poor antigen expression. Only in 1989, almost ten years after Ilana's first attempts and five years after Paul's successful demonstration that TIL could be grown from other tumors, was Jim Yang, one of the best scientists in my lab, able to grow TIL from the MCA-102 tumor. Jim, who later joined our senior staff, succeeded only because he believed firmly that it could be done and only after exhaustive experimentation and manipulation of cell-culturing techniques.

The failure to find TIL earlier demonstrates that experiments do not work; investigators make them work. And to do that they must believe in what they are doing. Had Ilana and I been convinced that we would find specific recognition and killing activity by T cells in tumors, we would have tried other tumors and other systems. Back then, I had not had enough confidence in the existence of these antigens to exhaust all possibilities before moving on.

Had we tried almost any other tumor in 1980, we would have succeeded. But at the time I had no reason to think that MCA-102 was any different from MCA-105. We had been testing many other hypotheses that had not worked and could not work because they were wrong. So we considered Ilana's failed search just another flawed hypothesis. Then the discovery of LAK diverted us. The particular choice of the MCA-102 tumor had cost us five years.

For decades most immunologists had believed that, regardless of animal data, human cancers did *not* have unique antigens that could enable the immune system to distinguish between cancerous and healthy cells. This was the nightmare that had haunted me for as long as I had pursued immunotherapy.

If these immunologists were right, any immunotherapy might have only limited potential. We might not be able to improve significantly upon LAK cells and IL-2. Without unique antigens for immune cells to recognize and attack, we would have no way of aiming weapons we developed specifically at our targets, specifically at cancer cells.

But if cancers did have unique antigens, it might be possible to design an entire next generation of medical weaponry and aim this weaponry at the cancer.

Now we could finally find out. We could ask the main question: Do human cancers have unique antigens?

Linda Muul is a Ph.D. scientist whom I brought in and asked to set up a lab that would prepare and harvest LAK cells solely for treating patients.

She did well but the more time she spent on these tasks—and she spent ten to twelve hours a day with technicians preparing LAK cells for patients while solving the production problems— the more frustrated she became. "I'm a scientist," she complained, "not a production foreman. If I had wanted to run a factory I'd have gotten an M.B.A. and made a lot more money."

She now had her chance to do science. I asked her to try to demonstrate that human tumors have unique antigens.

Linda took three vials of cryopreserved human melanoma from the freezer. (We freeze blood and tumor samples from all our immunotherapy patients at −180° centigrade; this provides us with material for experiments and also allows us to go back and cross-check any new findings with a large sample base.)

Paul grew TIL from this human tumor, then gave the TIL to Linda Muul. She tested the ability of the TIL to kill the tumor from which they were derived. *They worked, specifically. The patient's TIL killed the patient's own tumor.* Control cells were unharmed.

Linda then demonstrated unequivocally that human TIL were T cells. She also proved that these T cells specifically recognize antigens on their own tumor, and not on other tumors, and not on normal cells. These experiments had clarity, beauty, and simplicity.

Furthermore, the TIL maintained their killing activity when expanded 100,000-fold over a six-month period. Clearly we could grow them to huge numbers.

Kyogo Itoh and Charles Balch at M. D. Anderson Hospital in Houston also reported specific killing activity in human melanoma TIL. Soon many confirmatory reports appeared.

We had tried for five years to find lymphocytes that would recognize unique cancer antigens on human cancers. Now TIL cells had revealed their existence.

My old nightmare that cancers did not generate antigen, and that therefore immunotherapy could not work, was over.

Einstein once said, "The years of anxious searching in the dark and the final emergence into the light—only those who have experienced it can understand it."

CHAPTER TWENTY

On July 10, 1986, a year and a half after renewing our search for specific killers, we submitted our first paper on tumor-infiltrating lymphocytes to *Science*. As with all submissions, it was sent out to other scientists in the field for review. The significance of the paper was lost on none of them, and they returned it with their comments very quickly. Editors told us of its acceptance August 15 and published it a few weeks later. The last sentence of the paper observed: "Experiments with murine tumors, such as those described in this report, can provide the rationale for combining these therapeutic approaches to develop optimal combination immunotherapies for the treatment of cancer in humans."

We were already planning for our first patient and we had great hopes. A clinical protocol had been submitted for approval to NCI's Clinical Research Committee, and in the laboratory we had begun growing the tumor-infiltrating lymphocytes from several patients. Yet now, while we were moving so rapidly both in the lab and clinically, a heated attack on our clinical immunotherapy efforts was published. Oddly, the vehicle for this attack was another scientific report on our progress.

While we experimented with IL-2 and LAK, we had also been conducting clinical trials with IL-2 alone. Initially, we had administered the IL-2 cautiously. But when patients receiving both LAK and IL-2 began to respond to more aggressive treatment, we soon became more aggressive in the trials with IL-2 alone as well. Mike Lotze guided these trials, giving massive dosages of IL-2 alone three times a day, monitoring the patients closely, and pushing them to the limits of tolerance.

The new aggressiveness paid off. Of the first ten patients with advanced melanoma, all of whom were considered terminal, three responded. A sixty-two-year-old woman had had a primary tumor on her back and metastatic lesions in her lungs and pancreas; she was a partial responder. The second patient, a thirty-seven-year-old man, had lungs thick with tumor when he arrived, so thick he lacked the breath and energy to walk down the corridor. Lung X rays showed blocks of metastases clearly visible from across the room. There was nothing subtle about it. His liver and spleen also had metastatic deposits. These tumors all disappeared. His before-and-after lung X rays were dramatic and impressive. Yet most impressive was Nancy Burson, a thirty-six-year-old woman with three children who had endured a hemipelvectomy, losing her leg and half of her hip. She had been treated aggressively; amputations are uncommon with melanoma because when the disease spreads, it tends to go to all parts of the body. Now the disease had returned in her remaining thigh and her lungs. Doctors at Walter Reed Army Hospital had refused to give her a prosthesis because she had only a few months to live. That made her "very bitter," she later said. When she came to NIH, she was terrified and had given each of her children a piece of her jewelry to remember her by. After treatment with IL-2, she had a complete disappearance of her cancer, and five years later she shows no sign of disease.

After treating these ten patients with IL-2 alone, we analyzed the results in an article for *The Journal of the American Medical Association*, which published it in its December 13, 1986, issue. The journal also published an editorial about our therapy.

This editorial was a rebuke aimed directly at our work, and it got considerable attention. The editorial was written by Dr. Charles Moertel, a prominent oncologist at the Mayo Clinic. He did concede that our work "demonstrated that the lymphokines do have definite antineoplastic activity in human cancer, thus confirming a myriad of animal model studies."

But he argued that it was common for initial studies of new

treatments in only a few patients to claim great success even though these treatments "were subsequently discarded as ineffective."

He continued, arguing that the toxicities and expenses "are not balanced by any persuasive evidence of true net therapeutic gain. This specific treatment approach would not seem to merit further application in the compassionate management of patients with cancer."

His editorial did have an impact. A brief but intense flurry of stories about the controversy appeared in newspapers and on network newscasts. I had seen the responses in our patients. I knew I was correct. Yet I feared the publicity could slow our progress by discouraging hospitals from establishing immunotherapy programs, and by discouraging other scientists from working in the area.

The episode also caused me some personal pain because it happened to erupt the day before my daughter Rachel's Bat Mitzvah, and our family had gathered from around the world. I was saddened that this day did not belong entirely to Rachel.

Clinical data very soon seemed to resolve the controversy. On April 9, 1987, four months after the *JAMA* editorial, I published another article in *The New England Journal of Medicine*, summarizing our treatment of our first 157 patients with either LAK and IL-2 or IL-2 alone. All of these patients had advanced cancer and had failed other therapies. Forty-eight of them responded. Three of our patients died of treatment-related causes. (As we have gained experience, our mortality rate has declined dramatically. We push as hard as ever now and side effects can be severe— between one-quarter and one-third of our patients spend some time in the ICU—but, at this writing, we have treated more than 425 patients consecutively without a treatment-related death.)

The same issue of *The New England Journal* also included the first outside study, by Dr. William H. West, confirming our findings. He treated forty patients with LAK cells and IL-2; thirteen responded.

This time the *New England Journal* editor Arnold Relman commissioned an editorial to put the articles in perspective and, I believe, to reply to Moertel. Dr. John Durant, president of the Fox Chase Cancer Center in Philadelphia and one of the country's most respected oncologists, wrote this editorial and titled it "The End of the Beginning?"

Durant commented, "At the victorious conclusion of the North African campaign during the Second World War, Winston Churchill, in announcing its success to the British people, also evaluated its meaning. It was not the end of the war, nor was it the beginning of its end, but perhaps, he said, it was the end of the beginning, and so it proved to be. The observations reported by Rosenberg and West and their colleagues surely do not describe successful practical approaches ready for widespread application to the therapy of cancer patients. On the other hand, . . . perhaps we are at the end of the beginning of the search for successful immunotherapy for cancer."

It truly was the end of the beginning.

IL-2 was still considered experimental in the United States but the FDA soon put it and LAK in a special "Group C" category, to allow all comprehensive cancer centers in the United States to conduct clinical research with these therapies without special permission. More than thirty centers began such studies. In Europe IL-2 would soon be approved for general use.

By this time our own immunotherapy efforts were focusing on metastatic melanoma and kidney cancer, although we did treat other cancers. We chose to concentrate on those two because we were getting responses. Just as we studied only a few mouse tumor cell lines so we could limit variables and learn what did and did not work, these two cancers seemed ideal models in which to study, and try to improve, immunotherapy.

We have now treated more than 1,200 patients at NIH; these patients had failed to respond to all other therapies, had advanced cancer, and were considered terminal.

The response rate for melanoma patients given LAK plus IL-2

was approximately 20 percent. About one-half of those who responded at all to LAK plus IL-2 experienced a complete response, a complete disappearance of cancer.

About 20 percent of melanoma patients treated with IL-2 alone responded, but complete responses to IL-2 alone were unfortunately less common.

Thirty-five percent of patients with kidney cancer responded to LAK and IL-2, 22 percent to IL-2 alone. In both groups, about 10 percent of all patients treated had a complete disappearance of their cancer.

And a few weeks before the *JAMA* paper appeared, we treated our first patient with TIL.

We began a pilot study giving tumor-infiltrating lymphocytes to twelve patients. There were high hopes—these were the specific killing cells I had begun searching for ten years before—but there was also a logistical problem. Part of the preparation of human TIL involved the same techniques we had developed for murine experiments. We surgically removed a tumor. A lab technician then sliced the tumor into small pieces with a scalpel and placed the pieces in solution containing enzymes, which digested the slices and created a single cell suspension. IL-2 and nutrients were then added. Only those T cells that recognized tumor were sensitive to IL-2, and they grew. While they grew they killed the tumor cells. After three weeks the suspension contained only T lymphocytes.

But we could grow enough cells to treat mice in ten days. To grow enough TIL to treat humans, we had to expand the number of T cells found in the tumor by 10,000-fold. This expansion took four to six weeks and required constant attention—cells are living things, each one sensitive to its environment.

I asked Suzanne Topalian, a surgeon and a new fellow in the lab, to develop techniques for growing human TIL. By hand, manipulating cells in flasks and in 4" × 5" plastic plates divided up into twenty-four separate wells, she answered the necessary questions. After several months she developed a method that could grow T cells from 80 percent of human tumors. Then, with the help of industrial engineers from Du Pont and Fenwal, she began the development of a partly automated system.

It took us eight months to perform the pilot study to decide on the best way to administer the treatment. Extrapolating from the number of cells needed to cure mice, I initially intended to give at least 10 billion TIL to each patient. As the pilot study proceeded I soon raised this goal. First we surpassed the 100 billion cell figure. Suzanne Topalian later remarked, "Getting that high was like breaking the sound barrier. There were seventy-two separate bags we had to harvest. It took two days."

Then I raised our goal to treating each patient with 200 billion cells, enough to form a fist-size clump when concentrated, plus high-dose IL-2 and cyclophosphamide. We would give TIL almost exclusively to patients with melanoma. That would be the standard treatment we would evaluate.

The first five melanoma patients given this treatment all responded; their cancers shrank or disappeared entirely. We were extraordinarily excited. We thought we had really achieved something.

But as we treated many more patients, the response rate began to drop. Finally it settled at 40 percent, double the response rate with LAK and IL-2 or IL-2 alone. The best news in that figure was that patients who had failed to respond to LAK or IL-2 treatments responded to TIL at the same rate as patients who had never received any immunotherapy.

I tried to increase the effectiveness by creating synergies, adding other cytokines, subtracting cyclophosphamide, and making other adjustments. But the response rate continued at 40 percent.

TIL was a significant advance. When we published the results of the treatment of our first twenty-five patients in *The New England Journal of Medicine* in December 1988, it stimulated many other clinical and scientific groups to study human TIL.

Yet we could not grow TIL from every patient. And even when we could, 60 percent of our patients still failed to respond.

The pressure to improve what we had was intense. We knew our approach would work. *But the treatment wasn't working well enough*. For all the progress we had achieved, I felt frustrated and stalemated. I could see only two ways to end the stalemate.

One was to expand our knowledge base. We had to understand the basic mechanisms by which the lymphokines and immune cells acted so we could rationally design the approaches that would work best. There was, and is, an enormous amount of information—much of it at the level of basic science—that we simply did not know. Already we had started experimenting with other lymphokines besides IL-2. Now we started doing more. Jim Mulé found that IL-6 could cause tumor regression in mice and we later found that IL-7 could cause T cells to grow—and in some circumstances it made them grow better than IL-2. In the laboratory we took advantage of the ability of the interferons to increase cell surface antigens, and demonstrated that combinations of alpha-interferon and IL-2 would dramatically increase the antitumor activity of TIL—and this did lead to a clinical trial. We also became interested in a cytokine called tumor necrosis factor, known as TNF, which could make some tumors in mice melt away in hours. TNF seemed particularly promising to me, and we studied its mechanisms of action at a molecular and cellular level. And we began experimenting with different methods of using TIL to identify immune reactions against other cancers. Eventually Doug Schwartzentruber, a surgical fellow, would develop a technique to identify antigens on other tumors, including breast cancer and colon cancer—two particularly common and lethal cancers when they metastasize.

This first way to end the stalemate involved doing solid, methodical science, and showed promise. It also involved only incremental improvements. Science usually advances in such small increments.

But we needed to take a major step forward to improve the treatment—we needed to leap a chasm. One cannot leap a chasm in multiple small steps. The second way to end the stalemate involved such a leap.

. . .

One of the most important questions about TIL, and the very first one we addressed in patients, allowed me to consider such a leap. The question was whether TIL aggregated at tumor sites, whether they "trafficked" to cancer, or whether they simply circulated through the bloodstream and were randomly distributed through the body.

Our earlier studies of LAK cells had shown that these nonspecific killers did not traffic to tumors. Beth Fisher, one of our fellows, labeled TIL with indium-111, a radioactive isotope that was incorporated into the cell.

We infused these radioactive-labeled TIL into six patients. She evaluated the location of these cells on special radionuclide scans in NIH's nuclear medicine department.

Our third patient to receive the standard TIL treatment was the first one to whom we gave these cells. She was a forty-six-year-old woman with a large melanoma in her groin and another on her chest wall. The two tumor sites lit up on the nuclear scans. In six out of six patients, the TIL concentrated at tumor sites.

It was a crucial observation that would play a major role in our next strategic move—manipulating human genes.

This was the new direction that interested me the most.

PART FIVE

A NEW DIRECTION

On February 28, 1953, James Watson and Francis Crick discovered the structure of deoxyribonucleic acid, DNA, a structure with a significance impossible to miss. Its meaning leaped out at them instantly, and Watson later wrote in *The Double Helix*, "I felt somewhat queasy when Francis walked into the Eagle [pub] and told everyone within hearing distance that we had found the secret of life."

But there was truth in Crick's comment. DNA carries the genetic information for all forms of life. Overnight he and Watson had created the field of molecular biology—the nexus between physics and biology—and changed the direction of science.

Molecular biology had attracted me intellectually in graduate school, and I had known Watson, although only in the most passing manner. In the years since, the field had exploded. Probably at no time in history has any other area of knowledge moved as rapidly or as far in two decades. Recombinant IL-2 is only one of the fruits of this explosion. By the mid-1980s investigators were capable of genetically altering human cells as well.

To work our way through the five *if*s, we had searched for and found immune system cells that would kill cancer cells. All these immune cells existed in nature already.

The ability to isolate and manipulate genes meant that we were no longer limited to those cells that nature had provided to attack cancer. With genetic engineering, we could create cells with properties that had never existed before in the course of evolution.

The possibilities genetic engineering created were immense. It could open the door to an entirely new approach to treating not only cancer but all disease. This approach could dominate medicine in the twenty-first century.

Many diseases have some genetic component. Some, including sickle-cell anemia, are caused by a change in a single chemical base in DNA, a single character in a code that may run millions of characters long. Most genetically influenced diseases, however, are more complex. They are caused by flaws in several genes, a mix of genetics and environment, or both. Cancer is typical of such diseases. "Oncogenes" have been discovered, which can ignite cancerous growth, while other "suppressor" genes actually inhibit the transformation of normal cells into cancerous ones; the absence or presence of these genes may influence a person's susceptibility to cancer. And the Holy Grail of cancer research is a vaccine. Molecular biology might make it possible.

We began a series of experiments to insert foreign genes into TIL. If we succeeded, we intended to use TIL to introduce foreign genes into humans. It would be the first time in history this had occurred.

This approach was called gene therapy.

My efforts began in 1986, when I approached an outstanding scientist named Werner Green, one of the world's experts on IL-2. Green was then at NIH and is now at Duke University. He had the gene that coded for the production of the IL-2 receptor on T cells. (A gene resembles software written in a chemical code that stretches along part of the DNA molecule. The code orders the cell to produce one—and only one—protein. Humans are believed to have approximately 100,000 genes.)

I hoped to insert this gene into T cells and thus make them more effective cancer fighters. The logic was simple. IL-2 works indirectly against cancer by making T cells that recognize tumor antigens divide and grow.

Inserting a gene into a cell will make the cell produce protein it would not otherwise produce. If we inserted the gene for the

IL-2 receptor into T cells, they would produce many more IL-2 receptors on their cell surface than they did naturally. This would increase their sensitivity to IL-2 and could make them grow even more rapidly into much larger numbers. Cancer-killing T cells would then, I hoped, swarm through the body, seeking out and destroying cancer cells everywhere. This would be the Cinderella experiment I had dreamed of years before. An additional benefit might also come; it might allow us to use less IL-2 and thus cut down on toxicity.

I gave Werner Green TIL and he tried to insert the gene for the IL-2 receptor into them using a technique called calcium phosphate precipitation. The DNA one wants to insert is added to a solution that includes calcium phosphate and many target cells. The calcium phosphate forms a precipitate with the DNA that binds to the cell surface. The cell then absorbs the precipitate, and the DNA mixes with the cell's own genetic material. This is the single most common method of gene insertion but it is extremely inefficient. It rarely works on more than one in 100,000 cells. We made a few attempts but never succeeded in getting the gene into TIL.

About that time Michael Blaese and French Anderson approached me about using another avenue to gene therapy.

Most scientists choose problems to work on based on a combination of reasons. The most obvious are their own curiosity and the intellectual challenges a particular problem presents. They follow the problem wherever it leads, and often the insights and truths that emerge are far from their original pursuit. If they are experienced and talented, they will have an intuition about what questions are possible to answer, given the infrastructure of techniques and knowledge that has been developed. This, too, guides their choice of questions to study.

Other scientists, a minority, instead pick a goal that for intellectual or personal reasons they find so compelling that they pursue it almost obsessively. They persist even when the available technologies do not appear capable of yielding an answer. To these scientists, pursuing anything other than their original goal is a diversion. They force themselves to resist exploring what they consider side issues that they uncover and find exciting—and that another scientist might well consider more important—if they decide these approaches will not help them get closer to their goal.

From the beginning of my research I felt driven to look for new treatments for cancer. Similarly, for more than twenty years, French Anderson has devoted his energy toward developing gene therapy.

French is trim, as well groomed as a corporate lawyer. In his mid-fifties, French still has the litheness, movements, discipline, and goal-orientation of an athlete. Indeed, he holds a fifth-degree black belt in Tae Kwon Do, and once explained to a reporter that martial arts represented "a philosophy I was already practicing. The object is total control—control over mind and body, every part of your body. The object is to be totally relaxed, unless you're doing it in self-defense. Then you just explode."

As an undergraduate at Harvard, French was exposed to Jim Watson. He then went to England and worked in Francis Crick's lab, returned to the United States to finish medical school, and in 1965 came to NIH and worked under Marshall Nirenberg, a Nobel laureate who cracked the genetic code.

From the beginning French worked toward gene therapy. In the late 1970s he developed the technique of microinjection, in which DNA is physically injected into a single cell. He has said that even in his own lab the idea of microinjection was so ridiculed that he did the work at a microscope in his office, out of sight of others.

For all the usefulness of microinjection, one could not physically inject DNA, one cell at a time, into the millions of cells needed for gene therapy. Nor at that time could investigators easily clone a single human cell—grow millions of daughter cells from a single parent cell. So microinjection could not be used directly for gene therapy.

Many investigators were attacking the problem of inserting genes into large numbers of cells, and they developed several techniques that improved upon microinjection, including the calcium phosphate precipitation that Werner Green would try.

The most promising method was using retroviruses as a vehicle to carry genes into a cell. It was a way of using nature to change nature.

A virus cannot reproduce itself. Instead, it invades a cell and subverts the cell's machinery to produce new virus.

In most viruses, DNA carries genetic information. When these viruses invade a cell, the viral DNA sends direct orders to the cell's protein factories. The cell's machinery then makes viral proteins and new copies of the virus.

Retroviruses carry their genetic information in RNA, ribonucleic acid, which closely resembles DNA. When a retrovirus invades a cell, it must first transcribe its RNA into DNA, then have this DNA merge into the cell's own DNA. From then on, retroviral proteins are made in accordance with normal cell processes.

In the late 1970s and early 1980s, methods were developed to introduce a foreign gene into the RNA of a retrovirus. When the virus infected a cell, it carried these new genetic sequences into the cell along with its own.

Microinjection required the physical insertion of new DNA one cell at a time. Calcium phosphate precipitation succeeded in inserting a gene in at best one of every 100,000 cells.

A retrovirus could usually insert a gene into between one percent and 20 percent—sometimes more—of the cells exposed to it.

Adapting a retrovirus for use as a "vector"—a vector is any material containing DNA or RNA that is used to carry a gene into a cell—entirely changed the scenario for gene therapy.

But retroviruses are infectious agents. The AIDS virus is a retrovirus. Another retrovirus can cause leukemia. Other retroviruses may cause other diseases.

So the construction of a retroviral vector involved much more than just putting a desired new gene into it. A retrovirus used as a vector must be neutered; it must be impossible for the retrovirus to use the cell's machinery to replicate. Safety requires complex molecular manipulations and independent fail-safe mechanisms. A retroviral vector must be constructed in a way that allows it to infect a cell and then not produce any new virus. In the early 1980s, a research group including Richard Mulligan, a brilliant scientist at M.I.T. and one of the pioneers in developing retroviral vectors, found a way to do this.

While the technology of making vectors was progressing, other scientists were focusing on one specific disease of the blood called ADA deficiency, or severe combined immune deficiency, SCID, as a particularly good target for the first gene therapy. This is a rare immune system disease—so rare that there are only a few dozen victims in the entire world. It is caused by the failure of T cells to produce adenosine deaminase, or ADA; this failure in turn stems from a single defective gene. If a functioning copy of the ADA gene could be inserted into lymphocytes, the disease would be cured. Another advantage to ADA deficiency was it provided investigators with a large margin of error; a tiny amount of the enzyme could cure the disease, while a huge amount would not have harmful side effects.

French began to work with retroviral vectors around 1983. He was given the ADA gene by a scientist outside NIH who had cloned it.

French says that the night the ADA gene arrived, packed carefully in Styrofoam and dry ice, he told his wife, Kathryn, a prominent and skilled pediatric surgeon who is vice-chairman of surgery at Children's Hospital in Washington, that at last he was ready to start a gene therapy project involving ADA deficiency, but he knew little about the disease.

"Talk to Mike Blaese," she replied.

Mike Blaese is a large, bulky, broad-shouldered man, well over six feet and well over 200 pounds, who moves deliberately and with weight. He is smart, thoughtful, and a listener—a very good listener. Often people politely wait for someone else to finish so they can say what they want to say. Mike wants to listen, wants to hear ideas, and misses very little. He wants to do good things, as opposed to doing well, and he has no concern about credit. There is a solidness to him, a backbone he seems to provide to every project with which he is associated. His office and lab, like mine and French's, is in Building 10, the Clinical Center, on the NIH campus.

Mike is a pediatrician—French's wife knew him for that reason—with strong research skills and expertise in various immune deficiencies, particularly ADA deficiency. In 1984 French approached him. They immediately began a close collaboration with weekly joint lab meetings.

Initially French and Mike planned to insert the ADA gene into the bone marrow, which produces all blood cells including T cell precursors. That way the body itself could make T cells with a functioning ADA gene. They tried over and over and failed.

While French focused on making this system work, Mike began exploring alternatives. He had Ken Culver, a promising young investigator in his lab, try to put the gene directly into murine lymphocytes. It was a spectacular success. Mike knew of my work in detail. He suggested to French that they change course, remove T cells from a patient's body, insert the gene for ADA directly into the T cells, and reinfuse them into the patient. French said no.

Mike kept arguing with him. For three months French resisted. French says, "I was getting ready for another experiment in bone marrow. Mike said once again, as he had twenty times before, why don't we use lymphocytes? I don't know either how he got through to me or why I hadn't listened sooner. But for some reason I listened this time. All of a sudden I thought, 'My God! This will work!' "

In mid-March 1988, Mike Blaese walked three flights down the stairs from his office to come see me. We ran into each other in the corridor near my office—a community area by a blackboard on which announcements are written and by a grid of mailboxes. While people wandered by, checking their boxes for messages, we engaged in an intense conversation for twenty minutes. Mike already had a plan and he outlined it. I told him it made good sense. He suggested that he, French, and I get together to talk. I agreed.

. . .

On March 17, 1988, the three of us cleared off the pile of papers on the small conference table in my office. In a little over an hour we plotted a detailed path we would follow virtually without deviation for the next three years.

As in most good collaborations, we each brought something different to the table. I cared about helping people with cancer and knew T cells intimately. Mike cared about ADA and what it, as a model system, could teach him. French cared about the technology of gene therapy and knew more about retroviral vectors than either Mike or myself.

Our plan had to account for the politics of science as much as the science itself. Therefore we intended first to insert a harmless "marker" gene into TIL and infuse them into cancer patients.

The scientific justification for inserting the marker gene was the same one I had used in one of my earliest immunotherapy trials: to learn where the killer cells went in the body.

Labeling TIL with radioactive isotopes had allowed us to follow them and see that they trafficked to tumors. But the radioactive isotopes had taught us only a limited amount. The radioactivity can affect the cell, even kill it, and it wears off after a matter of days.

Marking the TIL with a gene would allow us to use biopsies and blood tests, in conjunction with a sophisticated DNA test called polymerase chain reaction, to detect one genetically transformed cell in one million. This was much greater sensitivity than we could achieve with the isotope. In addition, gene-marking would not harm the transformed T cell, nor interfere with its normal functioning, nor wear off. The gene would survive as long as the cell itself, or its daughter cells, survived.

There was a final advantage to starting with a marker gene. We were talking about manipulating genes in humans for the first time in history. By definition, the first time this occurred would be a historic event.

Years earlier a regulatory fortress had been erected to consider just this event; in the end we would have to pass through fifteen separate reviews by seven entirely different reviewing committees—as well as many subcommittees—each of which independently passed judgment on the scientific rationale, safety, and ethical ramifications of what we hoped to do.

Beginning with a marker gene was as conservative an approach—one by itself unlikely to raise safety or ethical concerns—as we could take, considering that it did involve genetic manipulation.

The goal each of us had was to insert therapeutic genes into TIL, which would help cure patients of disease. But almost any gene we might insert that could increase the TIL's ability to kill cancer cells would at least theoretically have some toxicity.

This potential toxicity would raise safety questions and make regulatory approval that much more difficult to get. Similarly, it would be more difficult to get approval if our first gene experiment involved the ADA gene because a partly effective and safe therapy for the disease already existed.

Using a marker gene first would not benefit the patient therapeutically, but it would narrow the focus of questions we would have to answer.

And using a marker gene would break the ice. We expected approval for subsequent genetic manipulations to come more easily than for the first one. After the marker gene experiments, Mike, French, and I planned to continue to work together, but we would function more independently. Mike and French would concentrate on inserting the ADA gene into lymphocytes and giving them to patients.

And I would insert into TIL one of several genes to enhance their ability to kill cancers, and give these transformed cells to patients.

We talked of all this in the intense hour on March 17. This meeting was a turning point for each of us. For that hour ideas about what milestones to set and how to reach them flowed with little effort. We became intoxicated by the possibilities of what this first gene manipulation could lead to. We all realized that what we were discussing was revolutionary, but it seemed so logical that—although we recognized succeeding would not be easy—we were confident we could do it.

When the meeting ended we knew specifically what our goals were. The different technologies required to insert genes into T cells already existed. This was no longer basic science. It was something we knew could be done. We had to do it.

CHAPTER TWENTY-TWO

Across the hall from my office is a large room crammed with bookshelves, scientific journals, a screen for slide presentations, X ray viewboxes, a microwave, hard chairs jammed close together, and a conference table so large that one must twist sideways to move between the chairs surrounding it and the wall.

It is not a comfortable room, but people who bring their own lunch eat there, and it is used for conferences. The discomfort has one advantage: It makes the room a good place to work when one wants to move through an agenda quickly and get blunt criticism. Beginning three weeks after French Anderson, Mike Blaese, and I first sat down, every Monday this room took on the feel of a war room. Everyone working on the project met there to review the preceding week's progress and plan experiments for the next week.

We were attempting to transform cells into ones with new properties nature had not given them. This would be a truly revolutionary treatment, yet many of the steps were relatively straightforward. We already knew how to take a wild, naturally occurring retrovirus, remove many of its own genes—so it could not reproduce itself—and make it into a retroviral vector that would carry a gene we wanted into a cell. We knew how to grow TIL. We knew how to insert the gene into the TIL. While we needed to refine our abilities to do these things, primarily we had to prove that all this could be done safely and reproducibly. And we had to prove it with enough rigor to withstand intense scrutiny from review committees concerned not only with the science but with political and ethical ramifications.

French, Mike, and I had laid out in our first meeting a five-step process that we would have to complete before beginning the clinical protocol. It was much more straightforward than the five *if*s.

First, we had to show that we could get the marker gene into TIL and show that it was actually being "expressed"—that the cell was making the protein that the gene coded for. Just getting the gene into the cell's own DNA was not enough. This step involved in vitro testing.

Second, we had to show that all other functions of the transformed TIL were not altered, nor unforeseen functions created. This step also involved in vitro activity and testing.

Third, we had to show that our system could work as predicted in animal models.

Fourth, we had to prove that the genetic transformation of the TIL and the use of the retroviral vector posed no threat to the patient.

Fifth, we had to demonstrate that the procedure posed no threat either to health care personnel or to society at large.

The overriding consideration was safety. There were several possible dangers.

A real, although very, very slight, risk existed that the gene insertion might cause the TIL to become cancerous. For this to happen, the gene we inserted would have to lodge at a precise spot in the cell's DNA to stimulate a natural gene in the cell, called an oncogene, which can cause cancer. Humans have three billion base pairs of DNA. This possibility was highly unlikely. But it was possible.

We could deal with this issue by testing the gene-modified TIL in the laboratory before infusing them into a patient. If any cells became cancerous, we would simply not administer them.

A second danger was potentially more serious. In the earliest days of recombinant DNA research, critics had worried that some nightmare "Andromeda strain," a new and dangerous life form, might escape from the laboratory. After several decades of absolutely safe research, this fear dissipated. But infecting humans with a laboratory-engineered retrovirus raised these concerns anew. It was theoretically possible for our crippled virus, which could not replicate itself, to somehow recombine inside the body with natural viruses to make a new virus that *could* replicate itself. The chances of this happening were extraordinarily slight. The retrovirus we were using was specifically engineered to make such a recombination extremely unlikely. We never saw it occur in any experiment in vitro, in mice, or in monkeys. But it was theoretically possible.

And there was another danger. Engineers working on state-of-the-art high-technology projects talk of "unk-unks," unknown unknowns. We were dealing with lives. Neither the review panels nor we could tolerate any unk-unks. We were not smart enough to predict with certainty the physiological effects of using the retroviral vector. We had to demonstrate that no unknown unknowns were hidden somewhere in the complex interactions between a virus and a living cell. Only many repeated experiments could demonstrate that an unknown unknown would not suddenly appear.

Every Monday at 3:00 P.M., working on questions simultaneously rather than sequentially, twenty to twenty-five people jammed the conference room to address these problems. At 4:30 each meeting ended promptly; at that time the Surgery Branch held weekly clinical conferences.

I was the principal investigator—it was a clinical protocol and we would be using TIL in my patients—but three entire labs were involved, along with Genetic Therapy Inc., GTI, a biotechnology company that French had helped set up. (A 1986 law, designed to encourage companies to commercialize scientific advances made in federal laboratories, allowed limited collaboration, and French had no ownership interest in GTI. I had no connection to GTI or any other company.) Each group had its own boss. We all knew what needed to be done, but scientists at NIH are not accustomed to coordinated research directed toward solving more engineering and practical challenges than scientific ones.

The room was small, stuffy, and hot—hot in every sense. There was pressure. None was ever explicitly stated or exerted. It did not have to be. At each meeting I went around the table, one person at a time, and asked whoever was responsible for a particular project to give a presentation about what he or she had done in the preceding week. Each of us explained to peers or more senior investigators what we were doing. Each week everyone was expected to have something new to say. At each meeting, progress was expected from everyone. *Have you advanced the goal in the past week? If not, why not? How did you design the experiment? Did you try this? Why not? Did you repeat the experiment? Did you see the article in the latest journal of . . . ?*

And each week we inched forward.

We divided the responsibilities. The marker gene we intended to insert had often been used in experiments by other investigators. It was a bacterial gene that made cells resistant to G-418, a variant of a little-used antibiotic called neomycin, and was called the neo gene. The goal was to infuse patients with TIL transformed by the insertion of this neo gene.

The retroviral vector that would carry this gene into TIL was a version of one developed by Eli Gilboa when he was at Princeton University and further modified to increase its safety by Dusty Miller at the Fred Hutchinson Cancer Center in Seattle. It was made for us by GTI. Having GTI supply the vector simplified meeting FDA mandates because the company, as any commercial entity would, designed its production process with FDA requirements in mind, something investigators at NIH could not easily do.

French's lab, especially Ken Cornetta and Rick Morgan, was responsible for developing sensitive assays to detect the vector and test it to guarantee that it did not contain any replication-competent virus—any viral particles that could reproduce themselves. This was crucial, since the vector was derived from a retrovirus that caused leukemia in mice. There was zero tolerance in the protocol for any viral particle capable of reproduction.

Attan Kasid and Paul Aebersold in my lab performed the actual transformation of human TIL. The procedure is simple in theory. A solution that contains the retroviral vector is mixed with a solution that contains the target cells; the transformation process is called "transduction." Yet much had to be worked out. Our first attempt to transduce human TIL with the neo gene was made on May 23, 1988. The attempt failed. But soon we succeeded. Transduced cells were given to Shoshana Morecki, a visiting fellow from Israel in my lab, who tested the functioning of these TIL.

Because of the repetitive nature of much of the work, to speed things I did something that I would never have done in my own lab. I often gave two people the same tasks. That way if one experiment went wrong for whatever reason—say, contamination—we would have data from another one available. If both worked, so much the better.

Competition and tension developed. Egos became involved. We were in a race, not with any outside group but simply to succeed, to get on with it. Some of our most difficult decisions involved determining when the proof was sufficient. Our goal was not only convincing ourselves of the reliability of a result, but also foreseeing any conceivable objections that a review group might raise. How much evidence was enough?

"It's time to declare success on that issue and move on," I said time after time. And everyone would be pleased to have moved one step closer to the goal.

But there was one important area in which we were having enormous difficulty finding success to declare.

Even before Mike Blaese had first approached me in the corridor, Ken Culver in his lab had genetically transformed a murine T-cell line—although these T cells were not TIL. Culver had inserted the neo gene with no problem and had performed studies with it. We anticipated little difficulty in getting genes into TIL. We were surprised. In repeated experiments we could not get the neo gene into mouse TIL. Neither could other investigators trying to do the same thing in other labs.

We gave fresh murine TIL to Culver. In the weekly meetings he initially reported encouraging results. But invariably the TIL died even before definitive tests could be completed. Tension developed over this problem, both directly attributable to these failures and over the different styles of some of the investigators.

My lab continued to be open, and all our information was available to outsiders. Not everyone agreed with this policy. Once, we thought we had discovered how to transduce mouse TIL and one participant in the weekly meetings, who was not from my lab, said, "Let's not let this get out that we know how to do it. We've got competitors out there."

There was a cold silence. Those from my lab looked at me. "My lab doesn't operate that way," I said.

If people in my lab felt free to give anyone who asked the answer, there was no point in the other labs' keeping secrets. They had no choice but to adhere to the same policy of openness. And it turned out we did not have the answer. We still could not transduce mouse TIL.

The weekly meetings became even more intense. We wanted the animal studies to support our protocol. We needed them. We expected the reviewers to insist on perfection before approving what would probably be the first time genetically transformed cells were given to a human being. We could easily get the gene into human TIL but neither we nor scientists elsewhere could insert genes into mouse TIL. I asked Jim Mulé of my group to try to do it. Jim could not succeed either. We are still trying.

NIH has thirteen quasi-independent institutes, of which NCI is one. Normally, a scientist at NIH must get approval of a clinical trial from the Investigative Review Board, the IRB, of his institute. If the trial involves administering a new drug, the FDA also must approve it. IRBs meet once a month, and the FDA must act within thirty days or permission is granted automatically. So the review process for most clinical protocols is brief and to the point.

Ours was not a normal protocol. The insertion of a gene into a patient exposed us not only to an extraordinary review process to ensure the safety of our effort but to bureaucratic turf wars and larger societal questions. We anticipated that the review process would be more difficult to overcome than the scientific problems. We were right.

Too often we were forced to turn our weekly meetings into a discussion of review stratagems instead of science. The first stratagem involved making the gene therapy protocol an addendum to our already-approved TIL protocol. This discouraged reviewers from raising questions about either TIL or IL-2, which had already been approved; the move drastically cut down on, but did not eliminate, what should have been irrelevant issues.

Difficulties came anyway, and they came quickly. On June 20, 1988, long before we had finished the scientific work, we made our first presentation to our first review panel, NCI's IRB, and the next day we had our first encounter with the IRB of French's institute. Both groups insisted we present more information on the safety of the experiments. Three weeks later, we presented our plans to the NIH Biosafety Committee, which judges whether recombinant DNA techniques are a risk to health care professionals or the public. It, too, insisted on more information.

Each of these review groups did, however, give us provisional approval. We would later have to return to each for final approval, but in the meantime we could proceed to the next step.

On July 29, we appeared before the gene therapy subcommittee of the Recombinant DNA Advisory Committee, the RAC.

Ever since scientists began working with recombinant DNA in the early 1970s, the public has been concerned. At first, laymen and some scientists feared the escape from laboratories of genetically altered life-forms that could live outside the lab. The city council in Cambridge, Massachusetts, passed ordinances limiting experiments at Harvard and MIT. But as DNA research proved safe, ethical issues involving human experiments and ultimately eugenics—attempts to improve the human race through genetic manipulation—replaced safety as the subject of debate.

Molecular biologists, motivated by concern about these issues and a desire to forestall legislation written by nonscientists, assembled in 1975 at the Asilomar Conference Center in California. Discussions there ultimately led to voluntary guidelines and regulations governing laboratory research, and to the creation of the Recombinant DNA Advisory Committee, which formally advises the director of NIH. The RAC includes not only scientists but lay representatives and ethicists; it later created a gene therapy subcommittee.

When the RAC was created, gene therapy was a distant dream. But in 1980 Dr. Martin Cline of UCLA, unable to get approval in the United States for what most scientists felt were ill-conceived clinical experiments, tried to perform one gene therapy experiment in Israel and one in Italy. Both experiments failed; in neither case could he insert the gene into the patient.

There were repercussions; one was the placing of severe limitations on Cline's ability to get future NIH grants. Also, scientists and laymen began to take seriously the possibility of gene therapy, and discussions involving scientists and ethicists began.

Virtually everyone agreed that changing genes in the germ line, i.e., in cells that transmit genes to offspring, is a dangerous manipulation under any circumstances. Even when the purpose of altering genes is to cure disease, this step would require extraordinary care because, given our current knowledge, it would be virtually impossible to predict all the effects on an offspring of changing even a single gene.

But there was far less of an ethical problem in manipulating genes in somatic cells—the kind we were working with—which do not bear on inheritance, particularly when the motivation was to save a life.

Putting genes into TIL fell into this category. We wanted to insert genes into the cells of a patient with advanced cancer. The cells could affect only that patient, a patient who was terminally ill and in dire need of treatment.

Yet our first presentation to the gene therapy subcommittee of the RAC did not go well.

The preceding year French Anderson and Mike Blaese had presented a preliminary plan for transducing bone marrow stem cells; the subcommittee had roundly criticized it, and soon thereafter French and Mike abandoned their efforts with bone marrow and approached me.

Our presentation ran into difficulties also. Two scientists on the panel who knew the field intimately and were early workers in gene therapy themselves raised the most questions. Over and over they pursued the issue of the safety of the retroviral vector.

We felt we had satisfied these concerns. The meeting grew heated. Leroy Walters, the chairman of the subcommittee, later conceded, "It got beyond an objective, cool, and rational discussion. . . . It's hard to see personalities get in the way of a supposedly objective review process. . . . A sense of competition did intrude, along with the despair of the investigators that nothing would ever be good enough to get through the subcommittee. . . . The investigators may have gotten the impression at least some members of the subcommittee would ask an infinite number of questions and try to stall the proposal forever."

Finally one member suggested that additional data be supplied and that when that data was presented, the subcommittee would be prepared to approve the protocol. That calmed things down.

On September 9, we wrote to the RAC subcommittee and provided additional information, but not all that had been requested.

We could not supply animal data about transformed mouse TIL because we still could not get the gene into mouse TIL. Jim Mulé experimented with ten different TIL cell lines. He tried TIL from four different mouse strains. He tried several different vectors, in addition to the one supplied by GTI. He tried different methods of inserting the gene, including calcium phosphate precipitation and electroporation. He tried variations of all these things. Nothing worked. Six different scientists in our three labs tried. No one succeeded.

We had put immense effort into this task. Clearly some unique properties made mouse TIL resistant to infection by the retroviral vector. Yet we could infect human TIL with the same vector.

All of us were aware the reviewers expected to see the results from mouse TIL experiments. We knew that several reviewers strongly opposed allowing any experiment to go forward without extensive animal studies; they feared that allowing us to perform a gene therapy experiment without them would set a precedent that later experimenters with genes would cite. Yet we would not be able to produce the animal data they wanted.

All of us knew of the reviewers' concerns and worried about them. But we could not spend more effort trying to do this; we wanted to treat patients and we could transduce human TIL. And Ken Culver had done extensive studies with mouse T cells that were not TIL.

Those studies would have to be good enough. Unhappily I said, "It's time to declare success and move on."

On October 3, we made our presentation to the full RAC, even though its subcommittee had not yet given its approval. But the RAC meets so rarely that if we had failed to make this presentation, our project would have been delayed for months. Still, some subcommittee members resented this. They believed we were trying to outflank them.

Several RAC members, especially some who served on the subcommittee, began to criticize the protocol. There was a hostile edge to their comments. They pressed for information we still could not provide on mouse TIL. And they continued to debate the theoretical possibilities of the retroviral vector causing cancer.

I tried to argue that this was a clinical situation, that we were dealing with cancer patients in desperate need of improved treatments, and that in a clinical situation one weighs risks and benefits. But I could not seem to make headway. The discussion continued over the most theoretical and hypothetical points. To me, some of it seemed like a discussion about angels, dances, and pins.

Finally, Bernard Davis, a highly respected Harvard scientist, made headway for me. He said it was ridiculous to argue over a highly theoretical risk of causing cancer in someone who already had advanced cancer and was dying. The committee was "nit-picking . . . The sicker the patient, the higher the risk you're willing to take. It is virtually not possible to have more risk than certain death."

It was a key moment. Discussion continued but one could feel sentiment shift in the room. RAC member Donald Carner moved that we be allowed to treat ten patients with life expectancies not to exceed ninety days. The motion was seconded. But more discussion, not a vote, followed. And the RAC adjourned for lunch.

During the break a special subcommittee was set up to discuss with me the informed consent form that we would have the patients read and sign. Writing the informed consent had been a Kafkaesque experience; all along the way different groups had wanted us to make changes in it, and then subsequent reviewers wanted us to change the changes. Now we were changing it again. But we agreed. The chairman gaveled the committee back into session.

There was still more discussion. Finally the RAC voted.

The protocol was approved by 16–5. Four of the five no votes came from gene therapy subcommittee members.

But we were joyous, exuberant. French organized a celebration dinner at a Chinese restaurant for everyone involved. He had waited for this moment much of his adult life. I expected the twenty or so people who had attended the weekly meetings to show up. About 100 did. All of GTI came. I had pictured the company as a handful of scientists and technicians. For the first time I realized the size of their effort. This dinner, too, had been prepared; there was a skit and laughter.

I felt distant from this celebration—not remote but a little apart. I have never been given to celebrating intermediate steps. We had accomplished nothing yet. We had only put ourselves in position to try to accomplish something.

And it turned out we had not even done that.

Legally the RAC is only an advisory committee to the NIH director. The director had to approve the experiment personally. We expected his approval and awaited it. But on October 18, James Wyngaarden said that he wasn't satisfied with a split vote. For an experiment that would for the first time transform the genetic makeup of a human, he wanted unanimity. And we had to provide more data to the subcommittee and get its approval.

On December 9, the gene therapy subcommittee approved the protocol 13–0. Later Wyngaarden conducted a mail ballot of the full RAC, seeking the unanimous approval he wanted. He got it, although one member abstained.

On January 19, 1989, we received approval from James Wyngaarden, director of NIH. The press release announcing his approval also noted that Frank Young, director of the FDA, had approved the protocol as well.

On January 30, 1989, at the next regularly scheduled RAC meeting, Jeremy Rifkin, an activist highly critical of DNA research, announced that he was filing suit to halt the experiment on the grounds of an inadequate review process.

At this RAC meeting, Rifkin filled the room with handicapped people—people in wheelchairs, blind people, people with other handicaps—and he showed *more* handicapped people on a videotape. In testimony he conceded that he was not opposed to our experiments per se, but to eugenics, and claimed that the pressure to correct genetic defects could lead to discrimination against the handicapped. He also hypothesized that manufacturers might require genetic alteration of workers before hiring them if a job exposed them to certain health risks.

Rifkin declared, "It is the first experiment in the world in which a foreign gene is to be placed into a human being. With this experiment we begin the whole era of human genetic engineering. . . . If we are not careful, we will find ourselves in a world where the disabled, minorities, and workers will be genetically engineered. . . . We will be back next time and the next time! . . .

We'll be back here every single time. You know we won't go away!"

The handicapped people he brought with him testified as well, saying much the same thing. All opposed allowing our work to proceed. It was a raucous, angry event, almost a demonstration. Politicians may see such scenes routinely; scientists do not.

I agree with Rifkin's opposition to eugenics. The idea of racial purification through any means is repugnant to me. When the RAC approved our protocol in October, one network news show flashed Hitler's face on the screen. The analogy stunned me. Both my parents were then living in Israel, and I was glad they had not seen it.

But Rifkin's arguments had nothing to do with treating a terminally ill cancer patient.

His suit charged that the final unanimous vote of the RAC to approve the protocol was made in a mail ballot rather than at a public hearing, and that this violated federal regulations. Yet before that mail ballot, the RAC had approved the protocol in a public meeting by 16–5. And the RAC is only an advisory group to the NIH director, who has the authority to overrule it.

Wyngaarden settled Rifkin's lawsuit quickly by agreeing to pay his legal expenses and reaffirming what was already so—that public concerns would be considered and votes would be taken publicly in all gene therapy trials. More than anything, I wanted to begin the clinical trials. Wyngaarden's course allowed us to proceed more rapidly.

We could now put a foreign gene into a human.

CHAPTER TWENTY-THREE

We had expected to treat our first patient with genetically modified TIL within a few days after getting final approval. We were eager to do so. Since TIL took four to six weeks to grow into the numbers we needed, even before we received approval we had begun transducing and testing cells of all TIL patients.

I had planned to await approval and then approach these patients, review the informed consent in detail, and ask if they would agree to participate in the gene study. If they refused, we would simply treat them with their normal, nontransduced TIL.

But we did not treat anyone soon. Instead, we were having problems.

The insertion of the gene began with the preparation of TIL. As with all TIL treatments, either I or a member of our surgical staff resected one or more tumors from the patient. Tumors have an unnatural, alien appearance; they are protuberant lumps wrapped in raw tissue. Melanomas are especially unnatural, even more alien to the tissue in which they are growing. Most tumors are yellow or pinkish, but for TIL we worked with melanomas, which are usually black. The black color is unrelieved, not shiny and reflective, like obsidian, but dull, as if it absorbs all things into itself. Yet from within this blackness we could grow lymphocytes that attacked cancer.

In the TIL lab, a technician carved away the normal tissue, cut the tumor into tiny fragments, and then placed them in solution with enzymes overnight, yielding a suspension of single cells. We used a gradient to remove dead cells, then began to grow what remained. After three weeks, when the T cells had killed all cancer cells and increased tenfold, we removed one-third of them and mixed them in solution with the retroviral vector. We also continued to grow the two-thirds of the T cells that we did not transduce. When the conditions were right, the retroviruses infected the T cells and thus inserted the marker gene into their DNA.

We succeeded in transducing TIL of two patients, but the transduced cultures became contaminated. The patients were treated with normal TIL. In two more patients, our tests did not show that we had met minimum standards of getting the gene into their TIL. They were treated with normal TIL. In one patient's TIL, we inserted the gene and her cells grew well. But she developed a brain metastasis before treatment. We were concerned that TIL therapy could be dangerous to people with brain mets, and had had discussions with the FDA about it. We did not treat her with TIL, normal or transduced. In two patients, we inserted the gene but their cells did not grow. They, too, received no TIL treatment at all.

We were only seeing one or two eligible patients a week, and sometimes none. At first weeks, then months, went by. Still we had not given anyone the gene-modified TIL.

The frustration in the lab became palpable. We had spent well over a year preparing to perform a single experiment. We had solved innumerable technical problems and made our way through a tortuous review process. We were finally ready. And now it seemed we were being thwarted by problems we felt we had already solved.

Each senior staff person in our lab, including myself, spends a two-month rotation each year overseeing the daily operation of the clinical service. My rotation for the year began May 1, 1989. At the time, several patients had transduced TIL growing in the lab. I hoped that, finally, one of them would be treated with their transformed cells, that, finally, we would transfer foreign genes into a human.

. . .

Lester Franks was a fifty-two-year-old truck driver from Indiana. He did not look like a truck driver; there was nothing burly about him. He did seem like a classic Midwesterner; lean, weathered, and straight, he was simple in his ways and exceptionally direct. He said little and was stoic about his disease. His great wish was to return to work; without work he felt unproductive and to him that meant his life had become meaningless. He was eager to try our most experimental therapies because that gave his life at least some meaning—what he was doing could teach us and help someone else. His wife supported him strongly.

He was one of those patients whose lives had been altered in an instant, and who had had little opportunity to adjust. Only a few months earlier, he had gone to a doctor, concerned about a mass on the left side of his neck. It was resected and proved to be melanoma. It was also extremely aggressive. The next month it recurred on his right side. A complete workup revealed that it had already spread to his spleen, liver, and lungs. He was sent to us.

We resected the right neck mass and used it to grow TIL. We then transduced his cells, as we were then doing with all TIL patients. But his transformed cells did not grow well and the tests to demonstrate that the neo gene had been inserted were equivocal. So we treated Mr. Franks with normal TIL.

Things did not start well for him. In a minor surgical procedure we put in a central line to gain access to his subclavian vein, a large vein in the chest that feeds directly into the heart. The line has three lumina—three different channels in the tube to allow us to administer different substances simultaneously and also to draw out blood for tests. This saves patients from being stuck with a needle each of the dozens of times we need samples. But he developed a pneumothorax and his lung collapsed; we had to put two chest tubes in. This was painful and uncomfortable. When he improved, we removed the tubes—too soon. We had to put a chest tube in again.

On April 29, he received his first infusion of normal TIL cells, while his gene-modified TIL continued to grow. After only three doses of IL-2, he became lethargic and confused, and his kidney and liver functions deteriorated. Jim Yang, one of the most aggressive doctors on my staff, wanted to stop his IL-2, although together we decided to push ahead. After two more doses of IL-2, he developed atrial fibrillation and his heart rate increased to 180. We stopped treatment. Mr. Franks was having a very difficult time.

I was, too.

For the second time in my life, a kidney stone was bothering me. A few days before beginning my clinical rotation, excruciating pain had sent me to the emergency room at Walter Reed Hospital in the middle of the night. They gave me morphine for the pain and intravenous fluids to wash the kidney stone away. I improved but a few days later the pain returned. On May 2, I took several bottles of intravenous fluid home, had Alice hook me up to an IV in our bedroom, and I took 1,500 ccs of fluid over two hours. I was not concerned, but Beth and Rachel were shocked to see me lying in bed with an IV in my arm. Although they had become almost accustomed to death from our conversations and from all the phone calls they had answered from desperate patients, they probably considered me invulnerable. All children consider their parents so. It made me think of Mr. Franks. He had young children.

I felt better soon. And Mr. Franks's transduced cells had started growing rapidly. We would soon have 100 billion. On May 13, we discharged him. If all went well, we would give him the gene-modified TIL on his second cycle of treatment in ten days.

But not all was going well. We had to prove that the marker gene had been inserted into the DNA of the cells. The first test was negative.

We prepared to repeat the test but first "selected" the cells. The marker gene made cells resistant to the antibiotic G-418. Adding G-418 to the cell culture would kill many normal cells but leave unharmed the transformed cells, thus increasing the percentage of transduced cells. The FDA would not allow us to treat patients with selected cells, but we could use them for tests. On May 15, we gave 100,000 selected cells to Attan Kasid, one of the molecular biologists in my lab, to test. It would take several days to perform the procedure.

Meanwhile another development occurred that pointed toward the future. I had an opening in my lab for a molecular biologist and interviewed Rena Zakut, an Israeli, for the position. She was very impressive and seemed the perfect person to work on a new project, a project I had been planning for over a year—cloning the gene for the tumor antigen that TIL recognized. If we could find this gene, we could begin developing a method to immunize patients against their own cancer. It would be a kind of cancer vaccine, and it might lead to other cancer vaccines.

I offered her the position and she accepted it.

For weeks, reporters had been calling NCI almost daily to find out when the first treatment of a patient with genetically modified cells would begin. Many reporters and photographers had requested to be present when genetically altered cells were first administered to a patient. They kept telling me it was a historic event and they wanted to record it. I refused all such requests. Then Jeremy Rifkin announced that he had settled his lawsuit and we would treat a patient the following week.

Everyone around me began to get excited. One could almost smell the excitement building. Reporters began calling constantly.

Then Mr. Franks's cells suddenly slowed their growth. They were living things, with all the unpredictability of any living organism. If they did not pick up again, we could not treat him. The entire lab stiffened. Daily counts of his cells quickly were communicated to everyone by those growing the TIL. It resembled listening to a radio for urgent information, but reports came only every twenty-four hours.

On May 17, another sudden jolt hit us when two FDA officials claimed that the agency had not formally approved the protocol. They insisted we answer more questions, which they submitted in writing. It shocked me and seemed more than simply unreasonable. We had already given the FDA mountains of data. Months earlier, an official press release had stated that FDA chief Frank Young had approved the protocol. The press had reported this approval. No one in the FDA had contradicted it. Now we had patients ready to go. But the FDA had the power.

On Thursday, May 18, I spent almost the whole day preparing the answers to the FDA's questions. French spent much of the day doing the same. We delineated precisely the ways in which we were planning to treat these first patients to eliminate the possibility of any later claims that we had been ambiguous. In most circumstances, I and all other NCI scientists do not speak directly to the FDA; instead, we deal with the FDA only through a special NCI section that works with the agency; our liaison official was Jay Greenblatt. I called him and said we needed a response from the agency immediately. If we had cells ready to give patients, we could not hold them while waiting for approval; the cells could lose their potency or become contaminated, hurting the patient's chances of responding. He promised to get an answer within twenty-four hours.

I was asked to attend a meeting in the NIH director's office to discuss responding to media inquiries. NIH's chief public affairs people represented Wyngaarden and told us he planned to issue an announcement when we had infused the cells.

In my entire professional life I had discussed experiments with reporters only after results had been published in a scientific journal, following peer review. Now we would not be doing that. We would not be discussing results at all, simply announcing that we had infused cells; we had no idea whether we could track the marked cells, or whether we had helped the patient. This experiment would be important only if it worked.

Wyngaarden's position was that he had to proceed publicly, that this was a historic event, and that it had already received tremendous public attention. The press had attended and written about meetings of the RAC and its gene therapy subcommittee. And we had come under attack from Rifkin. If we issued no announcement, the implication would be that we were hiding something. So Wyngaarden, as NIH director, would announce that the experiment had begun.

It was a political judgment. A day later another event occurred

287

that made me realize how the process had politicized me as well. On Friday an FDA official told me over the phone that we had FDA approval. I asked him if he minded if my secretary, Michelle Ragland, listened to the conversation to hear him say it. He agreed. Then I dictated a memo stating that Michelle and I had heard the FDA official give me oral approval. I signed the memo and asked her to sign, too. Doing this gave me an extremely uncomfortable feeling, almost a dirty feeling. It was not what scientists and doctors should be doing.

The process seemed to be changing me. All of the review panels and haggling over regulatory, not scientific, issues was changing me. In the past few months I had been talking about science and thinking about patients less and less, and had lost the total immersion in my work that I once had had and loved. It frightened me a little.

I thought of a man I knew who headed a major cancer center. He was a prominent and powerful doctor and scientist to whom laymen, journalists, politicians, and philanthropists listened. He was also a friend of my brother's. The three of us had gotten together once for dinner years earlier at Jerry's home, just as I was beginning my work with T cells. We talked about my hopes and what I was doing in the laboratory. My brother's friend was a big, robust, Irish fellow. He began to drink, and drank too much. Suddenly he became teary and burst out, his voice a mixture of anger, anguish, and torment, "I envy you! I used to do science, too! Then I started building buildings."

I wanted to get back to work.

On Saturday morning, the result was due from the test Attan Kasid had performed on Mr. Franks's DNA. Mike Blaese and I went looking for Attan and found him in the darkroom. He was just getting the result himself.

It was positive.

For the first time in weeks, maybe months, everything seemed to be clear. The regulators, the media, the lawsuit suddenly melted away. I had come to NIH to do science and to treat patients. Now I could get back to that.

For the first time it looked like we would give the cells to Mr. Franks, unless a last-minute catastrophe intervened.

We made the decision to proceed and to bring Mr. Franks into the hospital the next day.

Sunday afternoon, May 21, Mr. Franks returned. In the evening, we put in his central line. He was very nervous about the procedure because of the pneumothorax he had suffered in his earlier treatment. Under local anesthesia, we placed the line into his subclavian vein. This time it went well.

In the evening I sat down with him and his wife and reviewed the informed consent. Mr. Franks understood it perfectly. He seemed excited about being the first patient to receive foreign genes.

We were finally going to proceed. But I was still apprehensive that something would go wrong, that the cells might die or become contaminated and we would have to abort the treatment.

Sunday night I slept fitfully. In the hospital everyone seemed so excited that, although I tried to keep perspective, I could not help but be caught up in the mood. Infusing gene-modified TIL into Mr. Franks would open a door in medicine. The possibilities of gene therapy are extraordinary. Manipulating genes creates an entirely new and almost unlimited way to deal with disease that could change the way medicine is practiced in the twenty-first century.

At 6:00 A.M. the cell harvest for Mr. Franks began. In our sixth-floor lab, Kate Ottaway, a technician, began spinning down his cells to concentrate them from approximately 100 liters of solution into four 250-milliliter bags. I checked in. That process was going routinely.

There was only one final obstacle. We had to check the cells just before infusion to guarantee that they had not become contaminated with bacteria or fungus. Mr. Franks's cells were particularly vulnerable to contamination because I had purposely omitted a fungicide from the medium this time. In his first treatment cycle, Mr. Franks had developed side effects so quickly I thought the fungicide might have caused them. We had to stop administering IL-2. This time I wanted to give him massive doses of IL-2.

At 10:30 A.M. I got a call from the microbiology lab. The gram stain on his cells was negative. There was no contamination.

We were going to proceed.

I climbed the stairs from my second-floor office to the sixth-floor lab and picked up the first two bags of cells, then walked back down the stairs, down the corridor, and into the ICU. French and Mike Blaese were there, along with Ken Cornetta from French's lab, my surgical fellow, and two ICU nurses. One ICU nurse drew the required pretreatment blood sample through the central line, then hung one bag of cells.

At 10:47 A.M. on Monday, May 22, 1989, the cells began to drip into Mr. Franks's bloodstream. The new era had begun.

The treatment itself was anticlimactic. How often had we all seen an IV drip? But after a moment, Mr. Franks looked down at his arm and said, "Well there's no hair growing yet, so I guess it isn't working."

We all laughed.

I called NCI's press officer, Paul Van Nevel, and told him we had started. He relayed the information to Wyngaarden's office, and the announcement of the experiment went out from NIH to the press.

We drew more blood samples—as the drip was ending, three minutes after it ended, and one hour after. The samples were coded for later blinded testing, including tests for the genetically modified TIL.

I understood the historic nature of what we had done and was excited myself. Yet I was not as excited as French or Mike. We had known how to do this procedure for over a year; actually infusing his cells represented no technical advance at all. We had worked out the scientific problems over the preceding two years.

It did represent, however, the first time a foreign gene was inserted into a human. It symbolized the future.

Later that day Mr. Franks received two more bags of normal TIL. This emphasized to all of us that my goal was to help this cancer patient, and future cancer patients. Manipulating genes was useful to me only to the extent it furthered that goal.

Mr. Franks began to develop side effects from IL-2. We had included some in the bags of cells we had infused. He received a bolus infusion of IL-2 in the afternoon, and another at 3:00 A.M. I was checking him every few hours. After only two doses of IL-2 his bilirubin had risen to 3, indicating liver dysfunction. That was very high considering the little IL-2 he had received.

I decided to withhold more IL-2 and wait to see what happened. At 2:00 in the afternoon, his bilirubin was still climbing—now to 4.4.

He was excited, had watched the reports of himself on the television news—his confidentiality was protected and no one knew his name—but I could give him no more IL-2. I wondered whether the TIL would do him any good.

I was then on my clinical rotation, directly handling the moment-to-moment care of all the immunotherapy patients in the hospital. As we were treating Mr. Franks, the pressure grew. If anything had gone wrong with his therapy, regardless of whether it was related to the gene transfer or not, the repercussions could have been enormous. Nothing did go wrong with Mr. Franks. He went home on Friday, May 26.

Normally Saturday afternoons are my favorite time to work; in the quiet I go through the papers that have piled up over the course of the week. But without quite understanding why at the time, I needed some release. This Saturday, the day after Mr. Franks went home, I did something I have done perhaps only twice in the past ten years. I took off the entire day and watched Michael Jordan and the Chicago Bulls play the Detroit Pistons in an NBA play-off game. I love basketball and love watching Michael Jordan, but I agonized before turning to the game, not only because I was taking the time off but because I was not using it to be with my family. My enjoyment of the game was dulled; I kept thinking I should be doing something else.

I should have been. I needed that Saturday to help stay on top of lab work, which was moving at a rapid pace. During this year we would publish forty-eight papers, an extraordinary amount. IL-4 seemed suddenly promising. Jim Mulé had just found that IL-6 could make tumors regress. I was upgrading our capabilities in molecular biology and was beginning the search for the gene coding for the melanoma antigen. A dozen other lab issues demanded my attention.

So did extraneous issues—and for a change political developments proved useful to me. Senior people at the National Heart, Lung, and Blood Institute, French's institute, had apparently decided that NCI was getting too much credit for the gene research, and therefore wanted to pay for the retroviral vector. I had no objection; this would save my lab tens of thousands of dollars.

Since I was on the clinical rotation, I spent Tuesday and Thursday afternoons from noon to 5:00 or 6:00 seeing patients in the third-floor clinic. I would assess the results of therapy in anywhere from four to ten patients who had follow-up appointments. I would also usually evaluate four new patients, all with advanced cancer, who traveled from around the country to seek entry into our protocols.

New patients came to us only through referrals from their doctors, who had told them that conventional treatments could no longer help them. We were their last resort. In some cases, patients arrived knowing nothing of IL-2 or TIL; in others, patients knew of our work in detail and had demanded that their doctors call us. Whenever our work was in the press, the number of phone calls to our offices skyrocketed. Our research nurses did some screening; a doctor on the staff did more. To be accepted for treatment, patients had to fit into our experimental protocols. We offered entry into a research protocol to about three-quarters of the patients who came to the clinic. Almost all, after hearing a detailed description of IL-2's side effects and possible benefits, accepted it.

Clinic had changed little in the years since we began seeing responses, yet I never became accustomed to it.

There were painful ironies. One was that we had to reject some patients whose cancers were not advanced enough, who were not close enough to death. How could I tell a patient that we could treat him only when his tumors grew larger, that we needed more clearly defined tumor to accurately evaluate shrinkage if he or she responded?

I always had to walk a fine line between providing patients with hope while giving them a realistic view of what to expect from the treatment and their disease. One has to learn how to give bad news and provide hope at the same time. Many doctors cannot bring themselves even to use the word "cancer."

I had experienced the other side, the listening side, of this conversation myself. Several years ago Alice developed a ringing in her left ear. I had played the role of spouse, removing myself from the diagnostic process. One possible explanation was a brain tumor, but in discussing her case with me her physician could not say the word "cancer" and instead performed verbal gymnastics to avoid it, telling me Alice might have a "space-occupying lesion." I had felt terror waiting for test results. No abnormality was found.

It was impossible not to be consumed by clinic, saying yes or no to new patients, evaluating results in those we had treated. I remember many patients I was seeing at this time, but none better than the following two women.

One was sixty-four years old, and she had kidney cancer and lung metastases. Yet she had gone through worse, she told me. She was a survivor of the concentration camps. Numbers were tattooed on her arm. She showed me a letter from her sister, also a survivor of the camps, that said they would survive this, too. She and her husband cried when she showed me this letter. She did respond. Now, two and a half years later, her response is continuing and she lives a normal life.

Her response resonated in me and raised me up for a moment.

But the next moment I had to tell another woman who was thirty-two years old that her cancer progressed after one TIL treatment. She replied that she was putting her faith in God and abandoning all experimental therapies. She would come back to visit us healthy and whole, she promised. She never did.

Most patients did not respond. Inevitably came the question I had asked many times but could not answer, and which tore at me: Why had the therapy worked for some and not for others? How could we improve it?

We searched for other patients we could treat with gene-modified TIL. Finally our work began to go as close to smoothly as it can get.

On June 2, 1989, we treated our second patient, Kim Manafort. She was forty-two years old, an aerobics teacher, and as vigorous and upbeat as anyone we have ever treated. She developed melanoma on a finger, which was amputated. To her this was devastating. Her appearance meant much to her and, although virtually unnoticeable, she believed the loss of her finger marked her; she thought she would not be able to teach because students would constantly stare at her hand. She was angry at her doctor because her cancer spread despite the amputation. When we treated her she had large tumor masses at several locations.

On June 13, 1989, we treated our third patient, Richard Heat; on June 14, Michael Bartowski became our fourth; on July 21, our fifth patient was Edwina Schreiber. Meanwhile we continued to pursue laboratory research on other genes to insert.

The RAC had stipulated that all the patients receiving gene-modified TIL have a life expectancy of three months or less. No doctor can predict the life expectancy of a particular patient; one can speak only in probabilities. But all of the patients in the gene protocol had very advanced cancer and no alternative therapies.

On Mr. Franks's first follow-up visit, his lung lesions had shrunk, but not his liver lesions. His next follow-up, in November, revealed three brain metastases. We have treated very few patients with disease already spread to the brain and have seen no responses in brain metastases. This is probably because our treatment does not seem able to penetrate the blood-brain barrier; this barrier severely hinders substances in the blood, including immune system cells, from leaving the circulation and entering brain tissue.

We treated Mr. Franks's brain metastases with radiation and resected his spleen, which also had a lesion, and grew new TIL from it. Several patients have failed one TIL treatment and responded to a second. In January 1990, he received another infusion of TIL. His cancer did not respond. More metastases developed. He wanted to go home. In April, eleven months after his treatment with genetically transformed TIL, he died.

Kim Manafort had a 48 percent shrinkage of her tumor burden. Classification as a partial response requires a 50 percent shrinkage. She was carried in all our statistics as a failure.

But most patients in her condition would have died within a few months. Two and a half years later she is alive, active, and working again teaching aerobics, although her tumors have not disappeared.

Mr. Heat did respond, but the response lasted only a few months. When his disease began to progress, we re-treated him with TIL. This time he did not respond. He later died of his cancer.

Mr. Bartowski died several months after treatment. He showed no indications of any response.

The fifth patient was Ms. Schreiber.

She was a young woman in her late twenties, too frightened to travel here from Atlanta without her mother—her family had little money and we paid for her mother's ticket. She had come to us with thirty separate tumors riddling the soft tissues of her body and more tumors in her lungs. She had tumors in both tonsils. One tumor in her palate had pierced the mucosa, ulcerated, and was beginning to interfere with her swallowing. I considered it life-threatening and worried she could die before we had enough cells to treat her. We could buy time by irradiating her palate; radiation almost always shrinks a tumor temporarily. But radiation also suppresses the immune system; since the blood circulates through the body every fourteen seconds, virtually every lymphocyte in the body passes through the radiation field and is weakened. Instead we monitored her closely, ready to intervene if needed. Her cells grew rapidly and won the race. We gave her transduced TIL without having to give her radiation.

Her cancer disappeared completely. Two and a half years after her treatment she returned to the clinic for her most recent follow-up visit.

Her body still had surgical scars, and the cancer too had left a few marks, but they were only marks—small bluish spots on the inside of her arm, on the roof of her mouth, and at a few other sites, each one a stain of melanin left behind. The tumors in her tonsils had disappeared. The tumors in her chest, gone. In her breast, gone. In her lungs, gone. The ulcerating tumor in her palate, gone. The thirty other subcutaneous tumors carefully counted and measured, gone.

Two and a half years after treatment, when I confirmed that she is still a complete response, not only her face but her whole body shined with joy.

"Can I ask you a question?" she said.

"Of course."

"Instead of coming back every three months for a follow-up, can we make it every six months?"

I smiled. It marked her confidence. I agreed.

Even one patient like Edwina Schreiber was enough to keep me working at a breakneck pace.

Inserting the neo gene into the TIL of these patients had no impact on their treatment, nor was it designed to. It did successfully mark the TIL and allowed us to track the transduced cells. The marking proved that TIL were surviving in the patients. We consistently found these marked cells in the bloodstream of all patients for three weeks, and in at least some patients these cells survived for many months. Ethics forbade us from biopsying a tumor simply to get information if there was any risk of harming the patient, so we could not track TIL in tumors in all cases. But a tumor biopsy in Ms. Schreiber showed genetically modified TIL in the tumor nineteen days after infusion. Biopsies in Mr. Heat showed that genetically modified TIL were infiltrating his tumor sixty-four days after treatment. Later blood tests found cells with the neo gene in his bloodstream 189 days after treatment.

The marker gene proved that TIL were surviving in patients for long periods and trafficking to tumors.

But the most important findings of the experiment involved safety. Every single safety study performed on every single patient came out with a perfect result. In a *New England Journal* article, we detailed our findings in these first five patients, and we later inserted the neo gene into five more people with identical results: All safety tests were perfect.

Our study demonstrated that a retroviral vector could be used safely and effectively to insert foreign genes into patients. The neo gene could not help them in their fight against cancer.

But other genes could.

CHAPTER TWENTY-FOUR

In 1975, E. A. Carswell and Lloyd Old, two scientists at Memorial Sloan-Kettering Hospital in New York, first isolated a cytokine that had powerful killing activity against cancers—so powerful that they called it tumor necrosis factor. Within sixty minutes after injection, large tumors in the skin of mice began to necrose, and within twenty-four hours they were often completely destroyed.

The results were so dramatic that I found them difficult to credit fully until Tony Asher, a medical student in my lab, got the same results. TNF attacked tumors in two ways: by disrupting their blood supply, which killed them directly, and by regulating the immune response against them.

Yet TNF had shown no antitumor effects in humans. Several investigators had administered TNF alone to patients without result. Between November 1987 and September 1988 we also experimented with it, administering it intravenously with IL-2 to thirty-nine patients. We pushed hard—in fact harder than I had intended. The last patient treated required major support in our Intensive Care Unit and almost died. Even so, our trials did not find that TNF benefited the patients.

I believed that the results of these trials were disappointing because patients could not tolerate a TNF dosage large enough to be effective. On a per-weight basis, mice could tolerate fifty times more TNF than humans.

But TIL trafficked to tumors. Theoretically, if we put the gene for TNF into TIL, the TIL would aggregate at tumor sites and produce large amounts of TNF there. This would allow us to deliver enough TNF to tumors to kill them, while sparing the patient the toxic side effects that came from intravenous infusion.

To do this we needed retroviral vectors that would insert *two* genes into TIL, the TNF gene and the neo gene. We still needed the neo gene because it allowed us to select the transformed TIL easily.

For a vector to carry the TNF gene into TIL, I turned to Mike Kriegler, another Cetus scientist. Although I had not worked directly with him on IL-2, I had met him. Mike has three traits I value: He is smart, he is to the point, and he gets things done.

He was also one of the world's leading experts on TNF and had great expertise in retroviral vectors. In mid-1988, almost a year before we treated Mr. Franks and just before I ended the clinical trial giving TNF intravenously, Attan Kasid and I called and told him of our plans. He listened with enthusiasm and talked to company executives. I also spoke with senior executives. Cetus agreed to cooperate again.

Kriegler began sending us different vectors containing the TNF and neo genes. Attan began testing for the best one. He repeatedly transduced human TIL with each, then determined what percentage of cells included the exogenous gene and how much TNF the cells were actually producing. We kept no secrets. Attan reported each result at our weekly meetings, also attended by personnel from GTI, the company supplying us with retroviral vectors for our experiments with the neo gene. This caused conflict: GTI had also started preparing a retrovirus that would insert the TNF gene into TIL. They were eager for me to use their vector.

The potential importance of these vectors was immense. So was the field of gene therapy. If, instead of competing, all the scientists involved cooperated, I felt we could make rapid progress.

I made several unsuccessful attempts to bring the two groups together. My inability to do this was frustrating both because of the immediate problems it created and because of its implications for science in the age of biotechnology. I wanted to keep my relationships intact with both Cetus and GTI, not to mention French, a friend and a colleague. And I did not want to have to depend on one source.

I wanted the best vector, the best means of incorporating TNF into human T cells so I could give them to cancer patients. I decided to work with both companies.

By now, French, Mike, and I were moving down separate, if parallel, tracks. While I focused on getting ready for a clinical trial involving TIL into which the TNF gene had been inserted, French and Mike concentrated on preparing a clinical trial involving T cells transduced with the ADA gene. Although all three of us would be a part of both protocols and we continued to consult with each other, my lab did none of the science for the ADA project, nor did their labs do any for the TNF project. GTI provided all their retroviral vectors; both GTI and Cetus supplied mine.

If the tracks were parallel, if we were pushing both the science and the review process as hard as we could, neither protocol was speeding along them. Sunday afternoon, February 25, 1990, the three of us planned to spend the entire day in Mike's office to finish writing the ADA clinical protocol so we could meet a deadline for the first review. It turned into one of the most difficult and disturbing days of my career. That day I had other concerns.

My relationships with patients are often intense and close, but I almost never socialize outside the hospital with patients. There have been only two exceptions. One of these was a patient who had first come to the hospital two years earlier, shortly after his wife had died. He was sixty-six years old, had advanced kidney cancer, and was close to death himself; we gave him IL-2 alone and his cancer disappeared completely. An extraordinarily engaging person who had been a diplomat, he returned to an active life traveling around the world for pleasure and business. But now, two years later, his cancer had recurred; a large lesion was invading his intestine and causing a life-threatening bleed. He returned to the hospital and we again gave him IL-2, and then LAK cells plus IL-2. This time it put a great strain on his heart. He completed the treatment but did not recover well. His heart began to fail and I called in NIH cardiologists to work with me. Despite all our efforts, nothing we did seemed to strengthen his heart. That Sunday I was desperate myself, desperate for some way to save him. I could not find a way.

He died of congestive heart failure. The autopsy revealed that lymphocytes had infiltrated his heart muscle.

As I write this, his is the last treatment-related death from our immunotherapy protocols. His loss left me distraught. I was his doctor, yet impotent to help him. And he was dying alone, without family. His condition deteriorated so rapidly that neither his two children nor any other relative could return in time to say goodbye. Only I represented to him the world he lived in, and, though we had mutual friends and had gotten to know each other, I felt inadequate in that role as well.

That day I went back and forth between the ICU and Mike's office. The connection between the two was not lost on me. The urgency in me to move forward made me desperate, and in the wake of his death the delays of the review process seemed more agonizing than ever. In our marker gene experiment, we had made our first presentation to a review board on June 20, 1988, and had received approval on January 19, 1989—seven months almost to the day. This time the review process would take longer.

Our difficulties began even before my first submission of the TNF protocol, at a March 30, 1990, RAC meeting where we were seeking approval for the ADA gene clinical trials.

RAC members blistered the ADA protocol with criticism. The chief issue was the safety of the retrovirus used to insert the gene. Yet this was very similar to the retrovirus used in our first clinical trial with the neo gene. There was also another issue: a nongenetic treatment did exist for children with ADA deficiency. The patients we wanted to treat were already receiving it. But this treatment was unlikely to be of long-term benefit, while gene therapy was at least potentially a cure.

In the end, the RAC flatly rejected the ADA protocol, and even criticized as inadequate the internal NIH review process—the committees and subcommittees that had all independently approved it. This would have repercussions.

Unlike the marker gene or ADA, TNF itself could be toxic. That toxicity had prevented us from giving patients large doses intravenously. The whole point of inserting the TNF gene into TIL was to increase the production of TNF at tumor sites while sparing the rest of the body. But since TIL are live cells and they could increase in numbers inside the body—and all daughter cells of transduced TIL would also contain the exogenous TNF gene—at least in theory the experiment could prove dangerous to patients, raising a safety concern in addition to those of the retroviral vector itself. I anticipated a rigorous review process.

Still, we were not operating in the dark. Because normal TIL produced some TNF naturally and LAK cells produced even more, and because of our earlier protocol giving patients TNF intravenously, we had considerable experience with it, along with a large body of data on how much patients could tolerate.

I also planned to start giving patients only a small number of cells into which we had inserted the TNF gene, then gradually increase the number in subsequent infusions. The starting number of cells would produce no more than $1/100$ of the TNF dosage tolerated by man. It seemed to me that this was a sufficient margin to allow us to proceed safely.

On May 2, I made my first presentation of the TNF protocol before the NIH Institutional Biosafety Committee.

This committee had been stung by the RAC's criticism for approving the ADA experiment. It rejected the protocol and demanded more information on the structure of the retroviral vector and on human and mouse experiments with TNF.

The process went on and on like this, through each of the separate groups that had reviewed the other protocols. And each group demanded that all of its concerns be satisfied. Sometimes the discussions seemed interminable. During one RAC gene therapy subcommittee meeting, a lay member of the subcommittee, a nonscientist, broke into the debate: "There is another meeting going on down the hall, an AIDS meeting. If this study was for AIDS, people would be beating down the door telling us to approve it."

The subcommittee did approve it, 13–0. On July 31, 1990, the RAC itself voted unanimously to approve the TNF protocol. It also voted 16–1 to approve the ADA experiment.

Gerard McGarrity, chairman of the RAC, called the vote "a historic moment" and declared, "The field of medicine has been looking for this kind of therapy for a thousand years."

We began negotiating with the FDA.

The FDA approved the ADA protocol in September. On September 14, soon after permission was granted, a four-year-old girl was treated.

While I was an associate investigator on the protocol—Mike Blaese was the principal investigator—I was not involved with administering the treatment. Long before we received FDA approval I had planned to take my daughter Rachel, who was just entering her senior year in high school, to tour several New England colleges. Rather than reschedule her trip, we went as planned. It was an exciting time and while I loved being with Rachel, I missed the thrill of seeing the ADA treatment get started.

But the FDA withheld approval of the TNF protocol.

We anticipated that we would get permission momentarily. My lab began transducing cells of all our TIL patients, as we had done before for the marker gene. It took four to six weeks to grow TIL, and we wanted to be able treat a patient as soon as approval came.

It did not come.

From our first preliminary encounters in the spring until the end of September, through October, November, and into December, the FDA and I went back and forth. The agency was not satisfied with our safety studies, and we presented more and more data.

On November 13, the FDA approved the Cetus vector. But this approval did not end our discussions. It seemed to intensify them.

One issue was the GTI vector, which had not been approved. French was incensed. Although most of the safety tests had been conducted on cells transduced with the Cetus vector, the two vectors carried virtually identical genes. And before treating a patient, eleven different tests would still be performed to guarantee that the viral preparation was safe.

Another issue was the dosage schedule. I had intended to start with a small dosage of transformed TIL, one that had a safety factor of 100-fold for TNF tolerance. If there were no side effects, I expected to escalate the dosage to our standard treatment with 200 billion cells. But the FDA insisted that I lower the number of cells we could infuse by a factor of ten, increasing the safety factor to 1,000-fold. More important, the FDA refused to allow me to give any IL-2 to the first three patients. It was very unlikely that TIL without IL-2 could help a patient, especially in low dosage. We were giving cells to patients in urgent need of treatment; the FDA dosage schedule did not constitute treatment. I refused to agree. Our negotiations continued.

Scientific problems arose as well. November 30 marked four patients in a row into whose TIL we had failed to insert the TNF gene. The numbers of retrovirus in the solutions supplied by both GTI and Cetus were low, lower than they should be. And Cetus began having production difficulties. One of twenty bags of their supernatant containing the retroviral vector was found to be contaminated, and all twenty bags had to be discarded. Mike Kriegler told me it could take several months before FDA-mandated safety tests on a new batch were completed. We started transducing cells with the as-yet-unapproved GTI vector.

Alice later told me she had never seen me quite like this. I would come home discouraged and wake up discouraged. The science was not discouraging me. Science I could work at, dig away at, feel some control over. The regulatory process was what discouraged me. It sometimes seemed beyond my control.

The only bright spot was coaching our daughter Naomi's soccer team. She was nine years old and in the fifth grade, and I had coached her soccer team since she was in the first grade. Each Wednesday afternoon and Saturday morning for the weeks of the soccer season I would steal two hours for practice and games. This season we had not done well; we had scored only one goal and gone winless. But in the last game the team underwent a magical transformation. For the only time all year the passing plays we had practiced actually worked. We won 4–0. The thrill that victory gave me went beyond the game itself. It made no sense how much satisfaction I felt. For a day, my frustration eased—but only for a day.

In November Robert Antrim, a forty-two-year-old man who had been through much, came to the clinic for a follow-up evaluation. He was quiet, calm, and did not react when we told him his cancer had not responded to TIL. I suggested a new operation to harvest another tumor and try to grow TIL again. He agreed. As we did with all our TIL patients, we would try to transduce his cells with the TNF gene.

On December 17, I tried to talk Suzanne Marotto into returning for treatment with normal TIL. She was a thirty-year-old woman; her TIL cells had grown and were ready to be infused. She refused. We had resected a brain metastasis and she was receiving adjunct radiation therapy to her brain. I advised her that interrupting the radiation course to receive her cells was the best thing for her to do. She still refused, insisting that she would finish several more weeks of radiation therapy before returning. Exercising some control over her body—and over her treatment— was crucial to her dignity. And the idea of cancer growing in her brain terrified her. It was her worst nightmare. "Without my brain, I'm not anything," she told me. We did not treat her and had to freeze some of her cells. But we had put the TNF gene into another aliquot of her TIL. These transduced cells were growing, albeit slowly, and we kept them in culture.

I spent December 31, a Monday, on the phone with FDA

regulators—speaking with them myself rather than through NCI's liaison. It seemed that we were nearing agreement. I was not happy with it but I could live with it. The FDA would approve the GTI retroviral vector, but we had to start with a dosage of only 100 million cells and could not administer IL-2. This increased the safety factor from the 100-fold I had suggested to 10,000-fold. But we could escalate the number of cells rapidly, and if no side effects developed we could ultimately add IL-2. The agreement was not final but that day's conversations made clear that approval would come soon. If we treated a patient whose cells had been transduced by the Cetus vector, we could start with a larger number of cells without IL-2, but we had to escalate more slowly before finally being allowed to give IL-2 with the TIL.

I decided we would start with the cells of whichever patient was ready first, no matter which retroviral vector was used to transduce them.

CHAPTER TWENTY-FIVE

Every doctor would like to confront a sick patient, make a swift diagnosis, and provide a decisive treatment that cures. Sometimes this happens, but not often. More commonly, diseases and symptoms are poorly understood or effective treatments nonexistent. In those situations, the most important thing a doctor can do is listen and talk to the patient. This helps in making a diagnosis and choosing a treatment, and also allows the doctor and patient to form a bond that is part of the healing process. It is a bond that allows the doctor to provide comfort when he or she cannot cure.

There is a strangeness to this bond. It is balanced, but not equal. The patient trusts; the doctor accepts the trust, and with it also accepts responsibility.

This offering of trust and accepting of responsibility can take years to develop in most human relationships. But between a doctor and a desperate patient—as most of mine are—the exchange of trust and responsibility can occur in minutes.

When I was a resident, a wise surgeon told me that the patients who loved him the most were the ones who had endured the most difficult treatment courses. When patients did well, they were in and out of the hospital quickly, and on rounds he was in and out of their rooms and said little. But when something went wrong, he hovered over his patients, talked to them repeatedly, and they felt that he cared. When patients are very sick, the bond grips both doctor and patient and pulls them together.

All the patients I care for have difficult and often unsolvable problems. The more untried and experimental the treatment we offer, the more listening and talking I feel a need to do. The trust given and the responsibility accepted form strong bonds. Suzanne Marotto and Robert Antrim, and later Barbara Spengler, were to receive a treatment no one had ever before received and which we knew little about. We talked often. I came to know them and the bonds we formed were especially strong.

Suzanne—I call her and think of her as "Suzanne" now, no longer "Ms. Marotto"—grew up in Brooklyn, married, divorced, and followed her parents, who moved to a town near Scranton, Pennsylvania. She was feminine and olive-skinned, and she spoke with an oddly soft Brooklyn accent, if there can be such a thing, and her voice conveyed determination and enthusiasm in a way that made those listening to her determined and enthusiastic.

In June 1987, a few days from her twenty-seventh birthday, she noticed that a mole on her thigh had changed in size and color. Her doctor performed a wide excision. The diagnosis was melanoma. The lymph nodes in her groin were removed and two were positive. She underwent chemotherapy after the surgery and did well for two years. Then the tumor returned in her left axilla and in her skin and she was referred to us.

When we first admitted her, on August 20, 1989, she had eleven subcutaneous lesions. She entered a new experimental protocol that Mike Lotze was running and for which we had high hopes, and we gave her IL-4 intravenously.

Very quickly we saw how unusual her combination of timidity and tenacity was. If she seemed gentle and vulnerable on the one hand, she was relentless and dogged on the other. After the first dose of her second cycle of treatment, her blood pressure dropped into the 60s, her vision blurred, and she felt chest pain. She wanted to stop the treatment. Our patients always have this right, but we moved her to the ICU, talked to her, and reassured her that we would monitor her closely. She decided to continue. Once she made that decision she stuck with it through eleven additional doses. This was the highest escalation in the protocol.

Despite our hopes for IL-4, not a single patient receiving it responded. As soon as this became apparent, we offered Suzanne and the others treatment with IL-2. She took ten doses beginning November 8. But a lesion in her left adrenal gland progressed, liver metastases developed, and new subcutaneous lesions appeared; they now totaled twenty.

On January 22, 1990, we operated, removed her adrenal gland, and used the tumor in it to grow TIL. On March 2, she received this TIL treatment, along with IL-2 and also alpha-interferon. Her cells stopped growing, however, and in her second cycle we gave her only IL-2 and interferon.

She responded.

Her liver lesions shrank and so did many of her subcutaneous tumors. No new lesions appeared.

She was ecstatic. We were, also, and hopeful. She did well for almost seven months, but in the fall she developed severe abdominal pain. We operated on October 15.

Her entire right ovary was replaced by melanoma, and there were multiple small nodules—small black pellets, too small to appear on scans—throughout her abdomen. We removed her ovary and tried to grow TIL from it. Her cells would not grow. On November 1, we performed another TIL harvest, resecting several subcutaneous lesions and using them to grow the tumor-infiltrating lymphocytes. This time they did begin to grow. But an MRI scan of her brain revealed a large metastatic cancer in her occipital lobe. Suzanne was asymptomatic but the size of the tumor and the swelling around it could quickly make it life-threatening.

On November 9, our neurosurgeons operated and removed it. Back at home she began radiation to her brain. On November 27 and 28, we took an aliquot of her cells and transduced them, using both the Cetus and GTI vectors. In mid-December her nontransduced TIL were ready. It was then that she refused to come in for treatment. We had to freeze her TIL.

The sense that she had some control over her treatment and, more important, over her life mattered very much to her. After her operations she always wanted to see the tumor that was removed. She disliked general anesthesia, always fearing that she would go to sleep and not wake up. It seemed terrible to her, the idea of having made it through this far and dying like that.

So did the idea of an accidental death. She got frantic in cars, constantly telling drivers to slow down when they were not speeding, pushing her foot to the floor as if braking when they turned corners. These feelings represented her need to control *something* and were born of her anxiety. "When I drive myself, I'm fine," she told me. "I'm in control then." Once she said, "It's your body. You can't just tell a doctor, 'Do whatever you want.'"

Her desire to feel she had some control over what happened is common among my patients, but she carried this need further, was disturbed by the loss of any control. To her the worst part of receiving IL-2 was the confusion it caused. Most patients suffer little or no disorientation; in others it is severe. She recalled once one of the immunotherapy fellows asking her if she knew the time. "I was looking right at the clock," she later said. "I knew what it was. I couldn't say it. I hated that."

Despite all her efforts, her independence had gradually been taken from her. She told me once how much she had resented her old supervisor at work, who had insisted that she work full-time or not at all, and had refused to let her work part-time. Suzanne had wanted both the independence work gave her and the money. Her parents had gone into their savings to help her keep her own apartment, but she had had to give that up anyway and now lived with them. She still struggled to retain her independence, struggled with everything. What was especially unusual was that as her struggle with her disease dragged on, she grew stronger rather than weaker.

She was strong. She had endured so many procedures over so long a period that she had worn down those around her. She talked of a friend in her town who also had cancer. A boy, a man actually, in his mid-twenties. They did not hang out together but everyone knew about both of them. When either of them went anywhere, people stared. She got angry over it. It was a small town, she said, and some of the people had small minds. What was the big deal if she was wearing a turban to hide her hair loss?

Whose business was it? But the people kept staring. The boy didn't like it. He stopped going out.

You gotta fight, she told him. You gotta fight.

He was married and his wife was pregnant. He said he just wanted to live to see his baby. It was only a few months, then a few weeks, then a few days. His world was collapsing. People continued to talk, he and Suzanne linked together in people's minds. The baby was born, a daughter. He saw her, and died.

"I got so angry when he died," Suzanne said. "He just gave up. He could have kept fighting." She bunched her fists, went inside herself for a moment, then repeated, "He could have kept fighting."

When she entered the hospital in January, forty small tumors were growing on her body. Her father said she didn't used to be religious but had become so as her disease had progressed. She didn't get her religiosity from him, he said, adding that he felt some antagonism toward the church. But he understood what it has meant for Suzanne and would say nothing bad about the church to her. It gave her confidence. She kept pictures of saints near her bed. Once, driving home from NIH to Pennsylvania, Suzanne and her mother were convinced they saw a vision of the Virgin Mary. When Suzanne was admitted to the hospital this time she said, "All last year I said this would be the year of my miracle. This is the year everything would go away. I'm just so certain I'm going to get well."

Meanwhile her transduced cells grew, but with a terrible slowness.

On January 8, we finally got formal—but still provisional—FDA approval to use the GTI vector. We still had to answer additional questions. But we could proceed.

On January 9, it became clear that slow growth was not the only problem with Suzanne's transduced cells. They also were not making as much TNF as we had either hoped or expected.

In fact, other patients' transduced TIL were also not expressing the TNF gene very well. And we were still having difficulty getting the TNF gene into TIL in the first place.

I decided to have Patrick Hwu, a medical oncology fellow who had recently joined the lab, work on these problems with me. Patrick had tremendous energy, enthusiasm, and motivation, and was one of the night crew. He often worked all night, went home when everyone else arrived, slept for a few hours, and returned. We began to examine every aspect of this problem in detail. It was important and extraordinarily interesting. I did not want his intellectual curiosity to distract him from the immediate practical problem, however, and reminded him, "There's only one thing more important than understanding this, and that is getting it to work."

We began to spend inordinate amounts of time together, designing or reviewing experiments. Progress was slow, torturously slow.

Robert Antrim had a wife and two daughters, one twenty and one nine—the same ages as my oldest and youngest daughters. Forty-two years old, he described himself as a "realist." He said he had never seen a doctor before his cancer developed, but, "It's pretty much all I've done since. I take it all in stride."

He said this with enough conviction that one could almost believe him. He was the kind of person who does what has to be done, and, when there is nothing left to be done, he accepts. There was a roughness about him, and a ragged, touchy pride. A Vietnam veteran, he said, "I did my duty. I don't begrudge those who shirked theirs."

He enjoyed simple things. He liked to work with his hands. In the hospital he made leather wallets and credit-card cases for his family. One of his greatest pleasures was playing Frisbee. He loved to throw a Frisbee around and make it do tricks. He worked in the metropolitan Washington area and earlier had lived close to his job, but he could not tolerate what he termed the "concrete" of the city or the suburbs. So he moved to rural Virginia, beyond the reach of Washington and near the Shenandoah Valley. His land was up on a mountain, about the highest land in the area, he said, with a view of water. He was a hunter but now that he lived in the forest he no longer hunted. It was enough, he said, to be out there. He commuted almost 150 miles round-trip to his job fixing office building air conditioners, roofs, plumbing, and whatever—"Jack of all trades, master of none," as he put it. To him, the commute was just something a body did, the price of living where he wanted.

In March 1987, a melanoma was excised from the right occipital region of his scalp. In July, a neck mass was found; it, too, was excised. For two and a half years he did well. In February 1990, the cancer returned in his right groin. It was removed and he came to us.

We could not resect any of the tumors he then had in order to grow TIL, so he entered a randomized protocol comparing IL-2 and PEG-IL-2. (PEG-IL-2 is IL-2 bound with polyethylene glycol. We hoped it might cut down on many of the side effects. It did not.) He randomized to the regular IL-2 and began treatment on May 15, 1990.

In July, at his follow-up, we found progressive disease in his right groin and a new lesion in his knee. On July 30, we removed this new lesion and used it to grow TIL. In early September we treated him.

He did not respond. He took what he knew might be his last trip. A friend of his ran a construction company, had money, and took him to New Orleans. He seemed to view it as the last outing of his life. Then he returned to the hospital.

On November 28, 1990, we resected another tumor and grew TIL from it. These cells grew slowly, but on December 17 and 18 an aliquot was transduced with GTI's TNF vector.

Meanwhile the tumor in his groin was growing explosively, approaching the size of a grapefruit.

I began to think he would be the first patient to receive TIL transduced with the TNF gene, but on January 14, a test to detect the foreign DNA in his cells showed a very weak positive.

His cells' growth was slowing as well. Soon the cells stopped growing entirely.

Normally when this happened we discarded the cultures. Cells rarely began to grow again, and we had found that the older TIL were, the less effective they were. But I was desperate. I told the TIL lab to split the cultures, and, when that failed, to redouble the concentration of cells in each bag. I asked a technician to pull out every trick she had ever used or heard of to try to get these cells moving again.

"I'll rock them to sleep in my arms," she replied.

The cells did start growing again.

I was routinely arriving at the hospital early in the morning now, sometimes at 6:30, sometimes at 5:30. There was so much work to do. When I was a boy, no matter how early I rose, my father had always already left the house to open the luncheonette for those souls who either had worked all night but were not quite ready to go home, or who started work in the gloaming and sipped coffee silently at the counter. I never saw him those mornings, and he was both an aching absence and a constant presence. He knew what work was.

To my father, getting out early had been only a burden. Yet I liked it. There was something clean and empowering about starting the day then, with the sky just beginning to redden in the east. The morning was fresh and brittle with the January cold, so brittle the day seemed ready to crack. I felt I could crack it, and crack open the hours ahead, filling them with opportunity and newness.

Meanwhile, our luck began to improve. On Saturday, January 19, Attan Kasid showed me the results of his tests on the DNA of Antrim's and Marotto's TIL. Both were now a strong positive. The TNF gene was present in both.

But was the TNF being expressed? Were the cells actually making and secreting TNF? On Tuesday, January 22, in the evening, after Sue Schwarz had already gone home, I checked her just-completed assay of TNF production. Looking at the results I thought of the long trip Sue had made with me, beginning with my days as a resident in Boston; we were continuing into the future as well. The transduced cells from Antrim were making

168 picograms of TNF per one million cells in a twenty-four-hour period. The protocol required at least 100 picograms. Mr. Antrim's cells had been growing slowly, but they had grown.

Mr. Antrim looked like a go.

I knew French would want to know and called him immediately to tell him.

I then went to the TIL lab and advised Paul Aebersold, who ran the lab and had been keeping close watch on the cells himself, to get ready to prepare them for treatment. He smiled and said, "The tortoise did it."

On Saturday, January 26, I examined all the data on Suzanne Marotto's cells. They were still growing very slowly. We had performed seven assays for TNF production. The results varied widely, and the average was 141 picograms. But according to the latest test, her cells were making only 90 picograms of TNF, below the 100-picogram minimum. In order to treat her I would have to ask the FDA to accept an average.

I called Suzanne at her home. She was out, trying to remain active. To keep busy, she volunteered as a secretary in her local hospital, and also exercised at the gym to maintain her strength.

When she called back she told me that ten or twelve new nodules had appeared and she was worried, very worried.

Monday, January 28, I had to make a final decision. Would we treat these two patients with their genetically transformed lymphocytes or not?

Mr. Antrim's cells were 80 percent viable. Suzanne's cells were 75 percent viable. Both exceeded the FDA requirement of 70 percent viable cells. Still, neither patient's cells were growing at a pace that made me comfortable.

Normally we waited until we had at least 100 billion tumor-infiltrating lymphocytes before treating a patient, and we preferred to have 200 to 300 billion. These two patients had only about three billion transduced TIL.

But the FDA was requiring us to start treatment with a tiny number of cells—only 100 million—and increase the dosage very slowly. By the time we could give gene-modified TIL the same way we gave normal TIL, two months would pass.

Yet we had learned that the older the cells, the less effective they were. We could not grow 200 to 300 billion cells and simply keep them sitting in culture for two months. That would lessen the chances that they would help the patients. If we were to treat the first patients with potent TIL, we would have to juggle cell growth and treatment schedules and try to coordinate the two.

I was anxious to proceed. Since the RAC's approval on July 31, almost six months had passed. Even before final FDA approval, we had spent weeks trying to find a patient with transduced cells. It had been more difficult than we had expected. We were successfully transducing cells in only one out of five patients. In some cases after transduction, the cells did not grow. When they did grow, they did not always express the TNF gene. In other cases the molecular biology went perfectly, but the disease progressed too rapidly for us to treat the patient. Each day had brought another disappointment. Now, finally, we could treat Mr. Antrim and, if the FDA approved the averaging of TNF production figures, Ms. Marotto.

But considering the slow growth of their cells, was it in their best interests to proceed? What if their cells did not continue to grow until we could add IL-2? I spent a long hour alone in my office, pacing and staring and thinking, trying to reason through the dozens of elements involved, trying to create order in my mind and sort through probabilities and options. There was no way of predicting whether the cell growth would accelerate, lag, or stop. And their nontransduced TIL were growing no faster. Giving them the gene-modified TIL would not in any way withhold a potentially better treatment.

I made my decision. The room seemed to brighten physically. Finally.

I told the surgical resident to call both patients. I wanted them in the hospital that afternoon. We would run tests on them and put in their central lines. If the final tests produced the results we hoped for, we would treat Robert Antrim and Suzanne Marotto in the morning.

I prepared the certificates of analysis required for the FDA, detailing all the tests performed on the cells, then called our agency liaison, Jay Greenblatt, explained the situation with TNF production of Suzanne's cells, and asked him to find out if the FDA would accept averaging the assay results. I also told him that she and her family were arriving soon. I would not put them through any psychological stress while the FDA debated the question. I had to have an answer in an hour.

In less than an hour he called me back. The FDA approved.

That evening I reviewed the informed consent with Suzanne Marotto and her family, and with Robert Antrim and his wife. It was written plainly, and did not downplay the risks. I assured them that if they refused we would still treat them with something else. I told them they would be the first people ever to receive this treatment—our first attempt to develop gene therapy for cancer.

After answering their questions, I left each of them alone to discuss everything and decide whether to sign the consent or not.

Forty-five minutes later I returned. "Do you have any other questions?" I asked.

Neither did. They wanted to help cancer patients who would come after them, and they sensed that they would be part of the process that could open an entirely new door for medicine. This excited, even thrilled, them. And they believed that surely this great step into the future could help them. They signed the consent.

At 5:30 the next morning, January 29, 1991, I arrived at work, thinking of all that I had learned in the last twenty years, of how far we had come, of how little we still knew. Outside my office door, in the laboratory, Nick Restifo was sitting at a computer. Young, still in his twenties, Nick studied painting before turning to medical school and science; he had an artist's creativity and sensibility, an ability to see the world differently as well as relate parts to parts and to the whole. In science as in art, this ability matters at least as much as intelligence, maybe more so. I wished him good morning. He had been here all night and was focused on his data, consumed by it, and did not hear me. I watched him for a moment, remembering the exhilaration I had felt myself at his age when I worked through the night.

I walked down to the Intensive Care Unit and, without waking them, checked on Mr. Antrim and Suzanne. They were in the Intensive Care Unit only as a precaution and to allow us to monitor them carefully after we gave them their cells.

I had hopes for this therapy, great hopes, but then I had always had great hopes. But all the attention outside NIH—for weeks reporters had been calling me on a daily basis, wanting to know when this experimental therapy would begin—and most of the excitement inside it seemed focused on the giving of the cells. That bothered me. My brother had been cognizant of that when he told me that administering these cells might be significant historically and politically, but not scientifically. Now I feared he was right. Giving the cells did not matter; whether they worked mattered. Would they do the patients any good?

At 7:00, on rounds, I visited them in the ICU for the second time that morning and examined results from blood drawn at 4:30 A.M.

Mr. Antrim sat up and joked with us.

I looked at the numbers on his chart and for an instant I was frightened, then reason took command. The numbers from his latest blood test indicated two entirely unrelated life-threatening conditions. His blood sample had to have been contaminated with intravenous fluid; another blood test soon confirmed this. Suzanne, too, was fine, awake, alert, and eager for treatment.

I walked up to the sixth floor and oversaw the harvesting of the cells. Suzanne's were finished first; 100 million cells without IL-2 were suspended in a 250-milliliter bag of cloudy fluid, which I carried to the ICU.

Outside her room, I handed the bag to the nurse, who was one of the ICU's best, and I told him the precise timing of the many required blood tests.

When we walked into her room, she looked at the bag and smiled. The nurse hung the bag, then plugged it into the IV tubing and turned a toggle switch. The cells began to drip.

Less than half an hour later, Mr. Antrim received his cells, too.

CHAPTER TWENTY-SIX

Robert Antrim and Suzanne Marotto remained in the ICU. After the treatment with their genetically transformed cells, they were subjected to the most intrusive monitoring available and underwent continuous testing. I anxiously watched for any toxicity caused by the cells and checked on them every few hours. No evidence of a single side effect materialized. They received a second infusion, 300 million cells—still a tiny dose—without IL-2, at 10:00 A.M. on Friday, February 1. All again went perfectly. At 10:00 P.M. I returned to the hospital to check on them. They were doing so well that I decided to remove their central lines and allow them to go home the next morning.

They did. But Saturday at midnight Suzanne rushed back to the hospital, suffering from severe abdominal cramps. She was frightened and so was I, but the problem was quickly resolved and we sent her home again the next morning.

Monday evening she and Mr. Antrim returned to the hospital, and on Tuesday, February 5, both received a third infusion, one billion cells, still without IL-2.

Again there were no side effects of any kind. But their cells were not growing well. Neither were their normal, nontransformed TIL. We would soon run out of cells to give them.

On Friday, February 8, they received three billion cells but no IL-2. On Tuesday, February 12, we exhausted our supply of cells. Suzanne received 5.4 billion cells. Mr. Antrim received none. Their nontransduced TIL were so old and had been growing so poorly that I decided not to give them for treatment.

We failed to escalate to the point where we could give IL-2. The number of cells they received was pitifully small.

Suzanne said some of her tumors were shrinking but when I examined her, these changes were minimal. We would have to wait for a follow-up evaluation.

The interest from the national and international media was intense. On January 29, I had authorized the NCI press office to release the fact that we had treated the first patients—no names were used and their confidentiality was protected.

In the meantime Suzanne read about herself. *The New York Times* and other papers reported that she had only three months to live, based on the restriction from the RAC that we treat only patients with life expectancies of ninety days or less. How must it feel to read that you will die soon? I worried about this but she glanced at me and said with what seemed unconcerned annoyance, "I know I'm terminal, but three months? That's just a number. That doesn't mean anything. How do they know how long I can live?"

The follow-up evaluations were disheartening. Suzanne's tumors progressed. So did Mr. Antrim's. I had not expected anything different, considering they had received so little treatment. But we did not quit treating them. I decided that we would operate again on them, remove new tumors, and try to grow and transduce TIL once more. For each of them, this would mark our third attempt to treat them with TIL.

When we operated on Mr. Antrim and grew TIL this time, his cells grew well, although we failed to transduce them with the TNF vector. In April 1991, we treated him with these TIL. Even before he left the hospital, several of his newer nodules had disappeared, and the huge tumor in his groin had softened. I had never seen him so upbeat. For the first time I heard him talking about the future.

But I knew it was too soon to tell anything. On May 2, he

returned for his second cycle of TIL. As I walked down the corridor to examine him—one of those walks when I did not know what I would find—I held my breath and silently appealed to whatever forces governed the universe to let his tumors continue to shrink.

The tumors had returned.

One on his arm had completely disappeared during his first cycle; now, in the two weeks between cycles, it had grown back to a small bump. Several others that had shrunk earlier now also looked as large as they had ever been. The April TIL treatment had killed most of the tumor cells. But the few cells not killed were so virulent that in two weeks the tumors had grown back to their former size. I worried that these cells would very likely be invulnerable to this second cycle of TIL.

"Do they hurt, Mr. Antrim?" I asked.

"No, not bad, but I feel that little piercing they get when they start growing."

"Well, we'll have to attack them again with more TIL tomorrow, when we give you the second cycle."

"You got that right. Beat the hell out of them. Can't do nothing else."

I was trying to be hopeful. But for the first time, I feared Mr. Antrim had no hope.

A few weeks later he returned to the clinic. He had lost weight. His arms were thinner, everything about him was thinner. Yet his tumors had grown even more, as if all his weight was shifting from normal tissue to tumor. In a way, that was happening. Whenever he came to the hospital he always wore a cap, a different one every time. This time his cap said "South Carolina Gamecocks," and his T-shirt said "New Orleans." His younger daughter, Rebecca, came with him along with his wife. He had never brought his daughter before.

"I'm just waiting for a miracle now," he said.

I offered him another experimental therapy. I did not feel that it was likely to help him, but it would have no side effects at all. And it would let him know we would not abandon him.

He agreed to enter the protocol and received this medication as an outpatient, commuting four hours round-trip every other day. I offered to arrange his transportation to ease the strain. His wife declined, saying she wanted to drive him. I was not surprised. At this stage of the disease, the family often wants to get more involved. We began to increase his pain medication.

On August 5, 1991, Mr. Antrim died. His wife waited a day to notify us. Although she did not say it, I had the sense that she had delayed because she knew we would ask her if we could perform an autopsy. We wanted to learn, if we could, whether the gene-modified TIL remained in his body. I think she did not want to refuse our request. But she believed he had been through enough. Mr. Antrim had already been cremated before she called. I cannot say that he and I had become friends, but we shared something important—more than a scientific experiment. And I liked him very much.

I wished I had been able to give him TNF-transduced TIL in large quantities with IL-2. Perhaps it would have helped.

Suzanne Marotto had already been treated twice with TIL; the first treatment had generated a seven-month response and the second time was the gene therapy itself. In February we resected a third tumor and tried to grow TIL from it. The cells would not grow. She wanted us to try again. We operated a fourth time.

She then had more than sixty palpable tumors on her body. Yet her chief complaint concerned her appearance. Once she said, "I don't like the way my body looks. There are so many scars. That's why I'm going back to the gym." There was nothing superficial in her concern; it reflected how much she wanted to be normal.

Now, however, she felt pain in her back. Her mother said to me, "She's worried. She told me, 'Ma, I think this is bad.'"

In July we gave her TIL grown from this fourth operation. This time severe side effects developed. After only one dose of IL-2 her blood pressure plummeted and she became lethargic. We stopped the IL-2 immediately and gave her other treatment, but no matter what we tried she seemed only to sink.

I feared that she would die of the treatment. Her parents hovered around her. It was a remarkable family. Seeing her lying there under the covers, shaking, so like a little girl, her hair fuzzy but growing back from the earlier radiation therapy, a small dark spot on her lip, which in passing might seem to be a cold sore but which I knew was melanoma . . . The scene was so painful. And I thought of what she had said months before, that this would be the year of her miracle.

She recovered, but the treatment did no good. On her follow-up evaluation, we found two new brain metastases. Her cancer was mocking everything we tried, and mocking my efforts to offer some hope. She understood the significance. When I left her alone with her father, she cried.

Then she asked me if she could get on an airplane.

"Of course."

"A friend with a brain met can't."

"Yours are tiny. They are at the edge of what we can see. You have no symptoms."

She wanted to know because she wanted to go to Florida. There was a park where you could swim with dolphins.

I nodded and examined her. Her tumors had become larger now. She was still trying to look attractive anyway. Some were painful.

"How are you feeling?"

"Oh, great."

We talked about more therapy. Since her first encounter with cancer, she had received an incredible amount of treatment. At this stage even the toughest patients have said, *All right, enough. Leave me in peace.* Not Suzanne. She wanted us to perform another operation for another TIL harvest. After four operations and four failures with the same therapy, the last one of which almost killed her, she wanted to try again. Her tenacity was amazing.

There was another experimental gene therapy that we were

working on, a way to genetically modify tumors. It had not yet been formally approved, but I could ask for a compassionate exemption in her case. (The FDA sometimes allows experimental treatments, before they are completely reviewed, when there is a compelling medical need in an individual instance.) I mentioned this as a possible treatment.

Instantly she agreed and wanted to know when it might start, whether she should go to Florida first. We had more work to do first, I replied. She could travel if she wanted to. She could go to Florida.

But I did not think she ever would. I think that swimming with dolphins was a kind of vision she held out to herself; doing it would be admitting the end. This was not like a patient's desire to go to Europe. It was much deeper than that; it was communing with nature and going back to the sea. Where life began.

Suzanne Marotto and Robert Antrim were the first two patients to receive TNF-modified TIL. They were pioneers who helped both us and people who would follow. They opened the door a crack.

Yet neither one received the therapy as we intended to give it. Partly because of the slow pace of their cell growth, partly because of FDA restrictions, we could administer only a tiny dosage of cells and we could give no IL-2. My brother, knowing this, had told me that administering the gene-modified cells to them might be significant historically and politically, but not scientifically. I had hoped he was wrong. Unfortunately he was not. Neither Suzanne nor Mr. Antrim responded.

With these two patients we could make only a tentative first step into gene therapy. I had learned long ago that defeating cancer requires boldness.

Perhaps with our third patient we could be bold. Perhaps we could reach the point of administering IL-2 along with large numbers of cells. Perhaps the third patient would push the crack open wider.

Barbara Spengler was fifty-two years old when we met. She was a nurse, her father a dentist, one brother a physician. Yet she said that even in that milieu, "Where I grew up you didn't talk about cancer. You didn't mention the word."

She came from a small town in the Sierra foothills in California and now lived in San Francisco. Her view of the world was filtered through a prism of humor. She had never been religious but now joked, "I'm getting there. My sister-in-law is a born-again Catholic. In the last five or ten years she's become a zealot. We didn't have much in common, but I'm beginning to see her side."

Energetic, intelligent, and upbeat—and independent, clearly independent—there was something solid and unshakable about her. She was a woman who took control of her life after a divorce, consciously making decisive and determined choices about her future. She had completed four marathons and three triathlons and still ran despite her disease.

In July 1983, a lesion was resected from her calf. It was melanoma. Seven years later nodules appeared on her trunk. They were excised and proved to be lipomas—benign. In November 1990 she went to Paris with a friend; he was Irish, tough, and reliable. A partner in a small manufacturing company, he seemed solid, like her, the kind of person beside whom one would like to go into battle. On the trip he noticed more nodules on her flank and trunk. They did not hurt. When she returned home she had one of these biopsied. It was melanoma. The lesions were excised but very soon, in January 1991, new lesions appeared in her right anterior chest wall and her right axilla.

"The prognosis was very bleak," she recalled. "By then my boyfriend and I were pretty involved. He was going to either jump in with both feet or leave. He jumped in."

She was strong herself, never joined a support group, and was making many decisions about her own treatment. A daughter suggested she get a popular book on cancer by Dr. Bernie Siegel.

Ms. Spengler didn't like it: "My daughter and her husband

were English majors. They solve all their problems by buying a book. Siegel makes you feel as if you have control. He goes too far. It's almost as if it's your fault if you're sick."

On January 30, 1991, she went to the University of California at San Francisco, to a clinic that specialized in melanoma. A board of doctors discussed her case. Instead of offering therapy, they offered a pyschiatrist. She could try chemotherapy, but . . . Unsaid was the fact that no chemotherapy regimen yielded anything more than a respite of a few months. In passing, one doctor mentioned immunotherapy and told her a new IL-2 program was just starting in San Francisco. She spoke to the doctor running it, but she had to get all the required tests through her health maintenance organization.

That had been delicate all along. The HMO doctor in charge of her care had been supportive but told her the plan would not pay for many more of these tests, and that she had to go to an oncologist with the health plan. That meant chemotherapy. Her HMO doctor knew nothing about immunotherapy or NIH. The doctor who was setting up the IL-2 program referred her to NIH.

We saw her first on March 5, 1991, and harvested a tumor for TIL on March 12. In the four weeks between this harvest and her treatment, on April 11—with normal, not genetically modified, TIL—new lesions appeared. She had seventeen palpable nodules. She received a large dose of TIL: 300 billion cells along with eleven doses of high-dose IL-2.

She did not respond.

But we had transduced an aliquot of her TIL. These cells were not yet available in large enough numbers for treatment, but they were growing.

Her transduced TIL continued to grow. We were also selecting them. These cells contained both the TNF gene and the neo gene, which made the cells resistant to the antibiotic G-418. We added G-418 to the medium. The antibiotic killed many of the normal cells; the transduced cells grew well in it. Pat Hwu, working with John Yannelli, who had taken over responsibility for growing TIL, had painstakingly worked out the optimal conditions for selecting the TIL and growing them.

Earlier the FDA had refused to allow us to give selected cells. I sent them a detailed memo explaining all the difficulties we were having transducing lymphocytes and getting the gene to express itself, and asked again to use selected cells. On May 23, the FDA agreed.

Less than 5 percent of the cells Robert Antrim and Suzanne Marotto received contained the TNF gene. More than 50 percent of the cells Barbara Spengler would receive—if she agreed to try the therapy—contained it.

I approached her about becoming the third person to receive TNF-gene-modified TIL. In her case the treatment would disrupt her life. Because of the slow escalation of the dosage still required by the FDA, she would have to stay in the Washington area for six weeks. Yet she lived in San Francisco. Her friends and family were there. And despite her cancer, she was still working full-time. Did she want to try the gene therapy?

She immediately agreed and asked only one question: Her friend could not be with her the whole time. Should he come when it began?

I told her the beginning was almost certain to go very easily. If we treated her with IL-2, that could be rough. It would probably be better for him to wait until later.

On May 25, we began her treatment with the same dosage schedule the first two patients received. But her TIL grew better—much better. We gave her cells twice a week, tripling the number each time.

Her cells grew and kept growing. I became excited. And she moved closer and closer to being the first patient to receive TNF-transduced TIL and IL-2.

During her weeks here she became a tourist; her energy was unabated and she visited, it seemed, every museum or point of interest in the area. She visited many more places than I had ever been to.

On July 1, she received 100 billion transduced cells without IL-2. She did suffer fever and chills, common side effects that we first noticed more than ten years earlier, when we treated our first patient with pig lymphocytes. But these side effects were of little consequence.

Now the FDA allowed us to drop back by a factor of ten and add low-dose IL-2—one-quarter the IL-2 dose we usually gave with TIL.

On July 5, she received 11 billion cells and this IL-2 dosage. The FDA required us to wait at least three weeks and monitor all side effects before treating her again. No untoward side effects developed.

On August 5, she received 28 billion cells and low-dose IL-2. We waited again. Side effects remained minimal. While here, she became a grandmother. Her daughter was in constant touch with her during the birth and sent an hour-long videotape of the baby by Federal Express.

Now we had to wait for her cells to grow. On September 23, we gave her almost all the cells we had, 90 billion, and low-dose IL-2.

And we waited once more.

While she was in the hospital for her last treatment, I asked her what she thought was happening to the tumors. She laughed nervously and told me she thought they were going away. But she was afraid to say or even think that for fear it wasn't so. This was an unusual reaction; most patients allow their hope to influence their perceptions. Her reluctance to talk about her progress reflected her discipline and strength. But her tumors *were* going away.

When we started her treatment with transformed cells, she had thirty palpable lesions. We measured each one.

Even before she received her last dose of genetically modified TIL and IL-2, some of these tumors had disappeared. Others had shrunk substantially. None had grown. And no new ones had appeared. This shrinkage had already lasted more than a month. She was already judged a formal response.

We biopsied two of her remaining lesions. Pathologists found no viable tumor in either. All of the tumor was necrotic. Six years earlier the pathology report on Linda Granger's tumor had reached the same conclusion.

I was excited, but contained my excitement.

I did not know how long Barbara Spengler's response would last. I did not know if her tumors would continue to shrink. As I write this, eight months after her first treatment, her response is continuing and her tumors are continuing to shrink.

The results of treating one patient did not allow me to draw any conclusions. But I did know that we were just beginning with this effort. I did know that she responded. And I did know that we had pushed the door open firmly now.

E P I L O G U E

When I began my first efforts to manipulate the immune system, more than twenty years ago, I had no way of knowing whether this approach would ever help patients with cancer. My hypothesis—that the human immune system could attack cancer—was untested, and at the time I feared that it would fall victim to Thomas Huxley's observation on "the great tragedy of science: the slaying of an original beautiful hypothesis by an ugly fact."

My first attempts at immunotherapy—the transfusion of James DeAngelo's blood to an elderly veteran in 1968, the transfer of pig lymphocytes to Linda Karpaulis in 1976, and the very low doses of IL-2 we began to administer in 1983—marked a tentative reaching for clues to build upon. The consecutive deaths of seventy-six patients with advanced cancer, who came to me for help but for whom the therapy failed, caused me to have agonizing doubts about our efforts. When weighed against these deaths, no success in the laboratory was reassuring to me.

But on January 29, 1985, when Steve Ettinghausen knocked on the door to my office with the X ray that showed tumor shrinkage in James Jensen's lungs, and when fifteen days later Linda Granger returned to the clinic and all her cancers were disappearing, I knew that everything had changed. We had shown that the human immune system could be made to discriminate between healthy and cancerous cells, and to target, seek out, and kill cancer cells wherever they were in the body. Immunotherapy *could* stimulate the body's own defenses to fight, and even sometimes to defeat, cancer.

We have now treated more than 1,200 patients with advanced cancer using IL-2-based immunotherapies. All of these patients had already failed standard treatments. Most had kidney cancer or melanoma. In 10 percent of our patients with either of these two cancers, the cancer completely disappeared. An additional 15 percent of these patients showed significant partial responses to treatment. And about 40 percent of melanoma patients treated with TIL have responded to therapy. These responses have lasted as long as seven years and are continuing.

On January 16, 1992, an advisory committee of the Food and Drug Administration voted overwhelmingly to approve the use of recombinant interleukin-2 for patients with advanced kidney cancer. With that vote, immunotherapy took a major step toward joining surgery, radiation, and chemotherapy as an established treatment modality for cancer.

This marked the first approval in the United States of a treatment for cancer that acted solely through stimulating the patient's own immune system. It meant that IL-2 therapy would become generally available to patients in the United States. Soon hospitals across the country would be able to offer it. And approval for treatment of patients with melanoma should be considered soon.

But this was only a beginning.

Kidney cancer and melanoma are models from which we can learn. Now we are expanding upon these models. Recently we have found that at least some human breast and colon cancers, like melanoma and kidney cancers, express unique antigens. If antigens exist, logic suggests that the immune system can destroy these cancers as well. We are just beginning to explore this possibility both in the laboratory and in clinical trials. In the future we will test other cancers for unique antigens as well.

Immunotherapy can succeed. We continue to explore other ways to stimulate the immune system, both with and without IL-2. Other investigators around the world are now attempting to improve and extend the therapy's usefulness as well. Immunotherapy is maturing into a fully developed modality of treatment.

We have progressed far enough to see the promise of this treatment. I believe that in the future immunotherapy stands the best chance of any available treatment of having significant impact on patients with a wide variety of cancers, and, at least sometimes, curing the disease.

We have only begun.

Our immunotherapy with IL-2 and TIL led us on May 22, 1989, to insert a foreign gene into a human for the first time. This, and the gene therapies we later gave Suzanne Marotto, Robert Antrim, and Barbara Spengler, also marked a beginning.

Gene therapy has the potential to surpass, and in the next century conceivably replace, other forms of treatment. The door to gene therapy is not only open now, but on the other side of it work is exploding down a multiplicity of paths.

In our lab, the explosion of genetic research has led us to pursue the ultimate goal of an immunological approach to cancer: the development of a vaccine to prevent it. Vaccines work by exposing people to a disease antigen that stimulates a powerful immune response. Vaccination uses the disease to defeat the disease. If these kinds of approaches could be made to work, it might be possible someday to develop a vaccine to prevent cancer.

We have begun searching for a gene that codes for a protein that marks a cancer cell as foreign—a cancer antigen. In theory, this gene could be used to generate an immune response to the type of cancer from which it was isolated. Then immune cells capable of killing this cancer could lie in the body waiting to attack any such cells that become malignant.

We are concentrating on isolating the gene for a melanoma antigen. Investigators in other labs are also seeking this gene, especially Thierry Boon, a scientist in Belgium, who has recently identified several candidate genes.

Each human cell contains approximately 100,000 genes; finding the correct ones could take years, and years more to develop a vaccine. But it *is* possible.

In a first step toward developing genetically engineered cancer vaccines, we have already begun a new clinical trial that involves modifying the genes of the *cancer* itself so we can use them to immunize patients against their own disease. Experiments in mice, begun by other scientists and extended in our laboratory, showed that cytokine genes inserted into cancer cells made it easier for T cells to recognize the disease. And after the T cells recognized and killed the gene-modified cancer, they circulated throughout the body and attacked other cancers.

On October 8, 1991, two weeks after Barbara Spengler received her final dosage of gene-modified TIL, I treated the first patient in this protocol. He was a forty-six-year-old man and a surgeon. We had removed a tumor from him, inserted a gene into his *cancer* cells, and grown these cells in culture. I then injected them into his thigh. Three days later I administered the same therapy to a thirty-year-old woman.

By the end of 1994 I hope to treat fifty patients in each of the first two gene therapy protocols—the first with gene-modified TIL and the second with the gene-modified tumor cells. It will take that long before we can draw conclusions about the effectiveness of these treatments. But we have already started working in the laboratory to improve them.

And we are no longer alone in the clinical application of gene therapy. Here, too, work is exploding.

On September 9, 1991, the first patient outside NIH to receive foreign genes was given a marker gene at St. Jude's Children's Research Hospital in Memphis. Gene marker protocols are about to begin in Lyon, France, at Baylor University Medical Center, and M. D. Anderson Hospital in Houston, and at the University of Pittsburgh, where Mike Lotze is running this protocol; in 1990 he left my lab to create his own immunotherapy program. Proposals for trials have been made in Italy and Canada.

Dozens of other clinical protocols are being discussed: Many of these involve cancer but many more are directed at other diseases. One proposed treatment would insert genes aimed at lowering serum cholesterol. One would manipulate genes to treat cystic fibrosis. One would help evade the blood-brain barrier by using gene therapy to kill brain cancers. One would insert a gene for an enzyme lacking in young children who suffer from severe lung disease. One would try to prevent clogging of artificial blood vessels by lining them with gene-modified endothelial cells. One would interfere with the life cycle of the AIDS virus. One would treat muscular dystrophy by transplanting gene-modified muscle cells. One would treat certain eye diseases by inserting genes into the cornea. Even treatment of fetuses in utero is currently being considered.

In Britain, a government study has concluded that no serious ethical objections exist to pursuing gene therapy. China has established an advisory committee for gene therapy.

But if the potential of gene therapy extends far beyond the treatment of cancer, gene therapy seems particularly relevant to it. In cancer we face a disease that has evolved ways to circumvent the immune system. The immune system has failed to evolve ways to keep pace. But by manipulating genes we may be able to achieve what evolution has failed to do.

We have not cured cancer. We have not even cured melanoma or kidney cancer. But I believe we have made a start in a direction that holds immense promise.

If we have had more failures than successes, many people are alive who would not be alive without our treatment. If they are a minority of those we have treated, this minority speaks powerfully.

Linda Granger was the first patient to receive LAK cells and IL-2 in high doses. At the time, her body was riddled with cancer and another doctor at NIH had suggested she spend her last few months traveling in Europe. As I write this, seven years later, she is completely healthy with no sign of disease anywhere in her body. Her goal had always been to make admiral. Now she has authority over one of the largest naval bases in the world and her Navy career is back on track.

Nancy Burson lost a leg to cancer but the amputation did not help her. Another hospital refused to give her a prosthesis because her doctors did not believe she would live long enough to use it. She was one of the patients in the study showing that IL-2 alone could cause tumor regression. Today, five years later, she is healthy, with no sign of disease anywhere in her body.

Edwina Schreiber came to us with tumors in her lung, her palate, throughout the soft tissues of her body. She was one of the first patients to receive genetically transformed TIL in the marker gene trial. Two and a half years later she remains disease-free and is about to remarry.

I do not know yet whether Barbara Spengler will also mark a permanent first success for gene therapy. I hope so. If not, perhaps the next patient will.

I do not know whether either of the patients given genetically altered cancer cells will mark a first success of that therapy. I hope so. If not, perhaps the next patient will.

And if these efforts do not succeed, I believe that something will.

When we started we were looking for the slightest crack in the disease, a crack we could wedge open. Science works this way; one probes nature, finds an opening in it, and hopes the opening leads somewhere.

Now we have found new cracks, new weaknesses in the sheer and bleak stone face of cancer. We have wedged these cracks open. Now we are trying to widen them. And the hope, of course, is to burst through them.

Once, sitting in an examining room in the clinic with Suzanne Marotto and her father, reviewing what steps to take next, she told me, "It just hasn't clicked right yet. The right combination hasn't clicked in."

Twenty-four years ago James DeAngelo presented me with a puzzle in the emergency room of the veterans' hospital in West Roxbury, Massachusetts. I have not solved it yet. I may never solve it. But some very large pieces have been moved into place. And I am still searching.

ACKNOWLEDGMENTS

I am deeply grateful to the dedicated scientists, technicians, doctors, nurses, and support staff I have worked with at the National Institutes of Health. Only a few of the many people who made important contributions to our work are mentioned in this book.

Many people helped in the making of this book. Jay Acton helped with all of the arrangements and has provided wise council throughout its preparation. He has become a good friend and I owe him special thanks. My niece, May Wuthrich, discussed the concept of this book with me for several years and played an important part in my decision to undertake writing it.

Andrea Chambers, executive editor at G. P. Putnam's, edited this book. My coauthor, John Barry, and I would like to thank her for her critical comments, which led to improvements in virtually every aspect of the text. We are grateful to have worked with someone of her intellect and talents. Phyllis Grann, chairman and CEO of G. P. Putnam's, had an enthusiastic and clear vision of this book that has never wavered. Her wisdom and insights have helped shape it into its present form.

My family has always been extraordinarily supportive. My brother, Jerry, and my sister, Florence, bought me my first books and have always inspired me. My mother and father immigrated to this country from Poland. They had little formal education but were the wisest people I have known. My father died during the year I was writing this book and his memory is firmly with me. My mother lives in Israel. She read parts of the book and made many helpful comments. Her main criticism was that I dwell too much on my failures and not enough on my successes. But the balance is true and I left it as is.

My wife, Alice, lived through all of the work described in this book, with me. She has read each of the drafts and greatly improved them. She helps me in more ways than I can describe, and I simply feel lucky to be with her. My daughters, Beth, twenty, Rachel, eighteen, and Naomi, ten, grew up as I was doing this work. Each night at dinner they would hear me talk of my work, and from an early age they would answer the phone and take messages from worried patients. They have been patient with me and always seemed to understand why I had to do what I was doing.

Naomi was especially helpful to me in writing this book. When I was writing the epilogue she told me that it should be the only part of the book you *have* to read if you need to write a quick book report. I followed her advice. So if you have to write a book report and don't want to read the whole book, just read the epilogue.

Steven A. Rosenberg, M.D., Ph.D.

GLOSSARY

Antibody
a molecule produced by specialized lymphocytes; antibodies circulate in the blood and can combine with antigens

Antigen
a molecule that is recognized as foreign (nonself) and gives rise to an immune reaction (antibodies or immune cells)

Binding
the adherence of one structure to another (such as an antigen to its receptor or a killer cell to its target cell)

B Lymphocyte (B cell)
a lymphocyte that originates in the bone marrow and is involved in antibody production

Cancer
a disease characterized by uncontrolled cell growth and by the ability of cells to spread (metastasize) to other parts of the body

Cell line
cells that are grown continuously and for prolonged periods in the laboratory

Cytokine
a substance produced by a cell and that has an action on other cells (examples are interferon, interleukin-2, tumor necrosis factor)

DNA
deoxyribonucleic acid; the basic molecule of the genetic material made up of nucleotide bases and sugars; it is composed of two strands in a double helix that bind to each other

Expression

the ability of a gene to result in the production of the protein for which it codes

Gene

the smallest element of genetic material made of DNA; each gene codes for the production of a single protein

G-418

an antibiotic closely related to neomycin; cells that receive the neo gene are resistant to exposure to G-418

IL-2

see interleukin-2

Interferon

a molecule produced by cells (most often white blood cells) that can inhibit cell division and has a variety of effects on the immune system

Interleukin

a molecule produced by cells of the immune system that acts on other cells of the immune system

Interleukin-2 (IL-2)

a molecule produced by lymphocytes that causes other lymphocytes to grow (it has many other actions regulating the immune system)

in vitro

occurring in the laboratory in a test tube, flask, or other culture container

in vivo

occurring in a living animal

Killer Lymphocyte

a lymphocyte that can kill another cell

LAK Cell

see lymphokine-activated killer cell

Laparotomy

a surgical procedure involving the abdominal (belly) cavity

Lectin

a molecule capable of binding to and activating lymphocytes (causing them to grow or to secrete lymphokines)

Leukocyte

white blood cell

Leukopheresis

the process of removing leukocytes (white blood cells) from the blood and returning the rest of the blood to the patient; the patient's blood flows out of the body, through a machine, and back into the body

Lymphocyte

a type of white blood cell that plays a major role in immune reactions

Lymphokine

a cytokine (see above) produced by lymphocytes

Lymphokine-Activated Killer Cell (LAK cell)

a lymphocyte that has been exposed to IL-2 and develops the ability to kill cancer cells

Lysis

the act of killing cells

Melanoma

a type of cancer that starts in black moles in the skin

Metastasis

a cancer that has spread from its primary site to another part of the body

Murine

of mice

Neo Gene

a gene that codes for resistance to the antibiotics neomycin or G-418 (which is closely related to neomycin); cells containing this gene will not be killed when exposed to these antibiotics

Neomycin

an antibiotic similar to G-418; cells that receive the neo gene are resistant to exposure to neomycin or G-418

Pheresis

the process of removing one cell type from the blood and returning the rest of the blood to the patient (e.g., leukopheresis refers to removing leukocytes—white blood cells—from the blood)

Prognosis

the expected outcome of a disease

Protocol

a written plan that describes the exact treatment to be offered to a patient; in a randomized protocol the treatment alternatives are selected by chance

Reagent
any chemical or biological material used in experiments

Receptor
a molecule that is present on the surface of a cell that can bind to other molecules; binding to a receptor usually induces a change in the cell

Recombinant
refers to the splicing together of pieces of DNA; can be used to modify life forms or produce biologic molecules

Resect
to remove during a surgical operation

Retroviral vector
a retrovirus engineered in the laboratory to carry a specific gene into a cell

Retrovirus
a virus that contains RNA instead of DNA

RNA
ribonucleic acid; DNA codes for the production of RNA, which leads to the synthesis of proteins

Sarcoma
a cancer of the soft connective tissues of the body (such as fat, fibrous tissue, cartilage, or the lining of joints)

Selection
the process of exposing a cell population to a treatment that results in the isolation of cells bearing a particular functional gene (such as exposing a cell population to G-418 so that all cells not bearing the neo gene are killed)

Strain
a colony of mice bred by brother-sister matings over many generations so that all mice of the same sex are identical twins (all have the same genetic material)

Supernatant
the liquid remaining after the solid materials have been removed from a suspension

Thoracotomy
a surgical procedure involving the chest cavity

Thymus
an organ in the chest in which lymphocytes mature; immature lymphocytes mature in the thymus into T lymphocytes

TIL

see tumor-infiltrating lymphocyte

T Lymphocyte (T cell)

a lymphocyte that matures in the thymus and has the ability to recognize foreign substances (antigens)

TNF

see tumor necrosis factor

Transduction

the process of inserting a gene into a cell using a virus

Transfection

the process of inserting a gene into a cell by mechanical means such as electroporation (electric shock) or calcium phosphate precipitation (sedimenting the DNA onto the cell)

Transformed

changed in form or function usually by the modification or insertion of genetic material (such as the conversion of a normal cell to a cancer cell, or the insertion of a gene into a bacterial or mammalian cell to give it a new property)

Tumor-Infiltrating Lymphocyte (TIL)

a lymphocyte that invades into a tumor and can be grown from tumors using interleukin-2

Tumor Necrosis Factor (TNF)

a protein molecule made by cells of the immune system that has many actions, including the ability to interfere with the blood supply of tumors

Vector

a molecule or other structure (such as a virus) used to insert a gene into a cell

Virus

a tiny infectious particle that can reproduce only by invading host cells

INDEX

Heat, Richard, 294, 295, 297
Hellstrom, Ingegard, 58
Hellstrom, Karl, 58
Hodes, Rich, 82
Hoffman-La Roche, 153
Holtzman, Arnold, 148
Hopeland, Sheila, 160–61, 194
Hunter, John, 43–44
Hwu, Patrick, 312, 327

IL-2. *See* Interleukin-2.
Imaging techniques, 178
Immune response to cancer
  British Journal of Cancer article on,
    57–58
  stimulated in animals, 58
Immune system
  AIDS and, 19
  attack on own body by, 20
  bacteria and, 20, 59
  how it works, 18–20, 60
  screening done by, 19–20
  transplanted tissue and, 20
Immunosuppressive drugs, use of, 20
Immunotherapy
  future for, 331–36
  history of research on, 59
  how it works, 1–2
Indium-111, 125, 256
Interferon, alpha-, 149, 200–201, 255
Interleukin-2 (IL-2)
  creation of nonspecific killer cells
    without, 134
  discovery of, 79
  EL-4 and, 142
  future for, 331–36
  -grown lymphocytes infused into
    humans, 124–26
  half-life of, in humans, 171
  human tolerance for, 181
  infusion of natural, into humans,
    160–62, 171–72
  as an Investigative New Drug (IND),
    148

lectin-free, 108–10
making human, 99–100
making mouse, 94–95, 96–97
PEG-, 313
purifying large quantities of, 146–58
response rates for melanoma patients,
  252
response rates for patients with kidney
  cancer, 252
search for new sources of, 132–34
side effects, 180, 181, 182, 191, 194
steroids and, 177
survival time of, after infusion into an
  animal's blood, 132
used alone to treat tumors in humans,
  249–52
used alone to treat tumors in mice,
  142–44
used to grow mouse T cells, 81
Interleukin-2 (recombinant) (rIL-2)
  infused into humans, 177–82, 188–91,
    193, 194–96
  infused into mice, 164–65, 169–70
  made by bacteria, 154–55
Interleukin-2 (recombinant) and
    lymphokine-activated killer (LAK)
    cells
  failures with, 218–21, 228–32
  impact of infection, 230–31, 232
  infusion of, into humans, 194–96
  infusion of, into humans by bolus
    injections, 196, 199–217
  infusion of, into mice, 165–69, 175–76
  need for intubation, 206, 229
  outside study of, 251–52
  patient reactions to, 219–21, 235
  press reactions to, 233–38
  response rates for melanoma patients,
    252–53
  response rates for patients with kidney
    cancer, 252–53
  side effects of bolus injections, 203,
    204, 205–7, 209–10, 216, 217,
    232–33
  treatment-related death, 228–32, 236,
    237

348